W9-BSZ-272

Review Copy

Please submit two tear sheets of review.
With the compliments of

U.S. list price: $47.00

FUTURA PUBLISHING COMPANY, INC.
P.O. Box 418
135 Bedford Road
Armonk, NY 10504-0418 USA

CARDIOTHORACIC INTERRELATIONSHIPS IN CLINICAL PRACTICE

Edited by

Anthony M. Cosentino, M.D.

Clinical Professor of Medicine
University of California
San Francisco, CA
Director, Residency in Internal Medicine
St. Mary's Medical Center
San Francisco, CA
Chief, Division of Medicine
St. Mary's Medical Center
San Francisco, CA

Richard J. Martin, M.D.

Associate Professor of Medicine
University of Colorado Health Sciences Center
Denver, CO
Staff Physician
Department of Medicine
National Jewish Center for Immunology & Respiratory Medicine
Denver, CO

**Futura Publishing
Company, Inc.**
Armonk, NY

Library of Congress Cataloging-in-Publication Data

Cardiothoracic interrelationships in clinical practice / edited by
  Anthony M. Cosentino, Richard J. Martin.
       p.   cm.
    Includes bibliographical references and index.
    ISBN 0-87993-655-X
    1. Cardiopulmonary system—Pathophysiology.   2. Cardiopulmonary
system—Physiology.   I. Cosentino, Anthony M.   II. Martin, Richard J.
(Richard Jay), 1946– .
    [DNLM: 1. Lung Diseases—complications.   2. Lung Diseases—
physiopathology.   3. Lung—physiopathology.   4. Heart Diseases—
complications.   5. Heart Diseases—physiopathology.   6. Heart—
physiopathology.   WF 600 C2674 1996]
    RC702.C385 1996
    616.1′2—dc20
    DNLM/DLC
    for Library of Congress   96–38646
                                                                            CIP

Copyright © 1997
Futura Publishing Company, Inc.

Published by
Futura Publishing Company, Inc.
135 Bedford Road
Armonk, New York 10504-0418

LC#: 96-38646
ISBN #: 0-87993-655-X

Every effort has been made to ensure that the information in this book is as
up to date and as accurate as possible at the time of publication. However,
due to the constant developments in medicine, neither the author, nor the
editor, nor the publisher can accept any legal or any other responsibility for
any errors or omissions that may occur.

Printed in the United States of America.

This book is printed on acid-free paper.

Dedication

To the memory of Mike and Connie, with gratitude and love.
Mickey Cosentino

Contributors

David B. Badesch, M.D.   Assistant Professor of Medicine, Division of Pulmonary Sciences and Critical Care Medicine, Clinical Director, Pulmonary Hypertension Center, University of Colorado Health Sciences Center, Denver, CO.

Christopher A. Bailey, M.D.   Pulmonary Disease and Critical Care Section, University of Oklahoma College of Medicine and Veterans Affairs Medical Center, Oklahoma City, OK.

Thomas Corbridge, M.D.   Assistant Professor of Medicine, Director, Pulmonary Rehabilitation, Pulmonary Division, Department of Medicine, Northwestern University School of Medicine and the Rehabilitation Institute of Chicago, IL.

Anthony M. Cosentino, M.D.   Clinical Professor of Medicine, University of California, San Francisco, CA. Director, Residency in Internal Medicine, St. Mary's Medical Center, San Francisco, CA. Chief, Division of Medicine, St. Mary's Medical Center, San Francisco, CA.

Mark O. Farber, M.D.   Professor of Medicine, Indiana University School of Medicine and Roudebush DVA Medical Center, Pulmonary Section, Indianapolis, IN.

Barry A. Gray, M.D., Ph.D.   Professor of Medicine, The University of Oklahoma College of Medicine and Veterans Affairs Medical Center, Oklahoma City, OK.

P. Anthony Haddad, M.D.   Pulmonary Disease and Critical Care Section, University of Oklahoma College of Medicine and Veterans Affairs Medical Center, Oklahoma City, OK.

Jesse B. Hall, M.D.   Professor Medicine, Professor of Anesthesia and Critical Care, Director, Medical Intensive Care Unit, Section of Pulmonary and Critical Care Medicine, University of Chicago Hospitals and Clinics, Chicago, IL.

Michael A. Matthay, M.D.   Professor, Medicine and Anesthesia, Senior Member, CVRI, Associate Director, ICU, University of California, San Francisco, CA.

Richard A. Podolin, M.D.   Staff Physician, Department of Cardiovascular Medicine, St. Mary's Medical Center, San Francisco, CA.

Frederick A. Tibayan   Medical Student, Harvard Medical School, Boston, MA.

Donald L. Yakel Jr., M.D.   Fellow in Cardiovascular Medicine, St. Mary's Medical Center, San Francisco, CA.

Foreword

The heart and lungs share a common cavity bound by rib cage, intercostal muscles, and the diaphragm. That changes in intrathoracic pressures are responsible for inflation and deflation of the lungs is readily understood and accepted. Less apparent is the effect of lung inflation and lung mechanical properties on intrathoracic pressures and even less evident is the effect of intrathoracic pressures and lung inflation on cardiac performance and pulmonary blood flow.

As recently as the early and mid-1960s, cardiac and pulmonary physiology and pathophysiology were studied in a single laboratory. Investigators were interested in cardiopulmonary dysfunction. With the advent of coronary angiography the cardiopulmonary laboratory split and the study of heart and lung performance in many centers was performed by cardiologists and pneumologists in separate and distinct laboratories. Exercise testing in the pulmonary laboratory measured work load, ventilation, oxygen consumption, and pulse rate. The emphasis was on mechanism of dyspnea. Exercise protocols in the cardiology laboratory were designed to detect myocardial ischemia.

At an even more clinical level in the mid-1960s, a critical care unit in all probability included respiratory failure, cardiogenic shock, and postoperative cardiac surgery. The "players" included cardiologists, anesthesiologists, and new breed pulmonary physicians. Gradually these disciplines became more narrowly specialized and patient care became further fragmented.

Meanwhile a wealth of clinical observations and data have accumulated but all too often without unifying concepts. A few examples should make the point. Closed chest cardiac compression was practiced for almost 30 years before someone asked about the mechanism of blood flow and the relationship to intrathoracic pressure. "P" pulmonale and a rightward axis shift during an acute asthmatic attack is not infrequent. Why? Equally intriguing are patients in cardiogenic pulmonary edema who during mechanical ventilation may experience an increase in cardiac output with application of PEEP.

The heart and lung share the chest cavity. Just as changes in intrathoracic pressure affect lung function so too may these alterations in pressure affect cardiac performance and often in a manner one might not predict.

It is the purpose of this book to review what is known about cardiothoracic interrelationships both in normal and abnormal states. I hope the material will be informative and intellectually stimulating for those who manage patients with cardiopulmonary dysfunction.

Anthony M. Cosentino, M.D.
San Francisco, CA

Preface

Dr. Anthony Cosentino has formulated an intriguing textbook on cardiothoracic relations in health and disease, with the major emphasis on the seldom addressed and often underappreciated influence of chest pressure and lung mechanics on the hemodynamic performance of the heart and pulmonary circulation. This obligatory linking of ventilatory properties with cardiovascular function in the thoracic cage are intricately delineated in the scintillating opening chapter on basic and applied physiology by Dr. Cosentino.

The mechanisms responsible for the formulation and resolution of pulmonary edema are next considered by Drs. Matthay and Tibayan. Both the etiologies of high pressure and/or increased permeability are depicted, and new data on the processes of alveolar fluid clearance are carefully examined. Then the cardiothoracic interactions constituting the modality of external cardiopulmonary resuscitation (CPR) are evaluated by Drs. Donald Yakel and Richard Podolin. While two contrasting mechanisms of CPR have emerged, the thoracic pump and the cardiac pump theories, both systems appear operative and successful CPR may actually require induced ventricular contraction.

Drs. P. Haddad, C. Bailey and Barry Gray provide an extensive treatise on the interdependence of heart and lung function in cardiogenic pulmonary edema. The pulmonary abnormalities in restrictive function, airway obstruction, respiratory muscle function, gas exchange, vascular compliance and circulatory distribution that comprise the congestive heart failure (CHF) state are critically defined. In regard to ventilatory therapy in CHF, besides the ability to sustain life and enhance lung function, positive pressure ventilation improves left ventricular (LV) performance by reducing excessive end-diastolic volume (preload) and end-systolic volume (afterload) and may result in an increase in cardiac output.

The chapter by Dr. David Badesch on cardiothoracic interactions relative to pulmonary blood flow and cardiac performance includes descriptions of the effects of intrapleural pressure on LV function; the mechanisms of heart disease and pulmonary hypertension on pulmonary blood flow; and the influence of right ventricle (RV) function on LV performance. Drs. Thomas Corbridge and Jesse Hall then discuss the occurrence, mechanisms, consequences and therapy of pulmonary hypertension in status asthmaticus.

The subject of cor pulmonale is approached in two sections. In the first part, Dr. Anthony Cosentino eloquently assesses the identification and pathophysiology with particular attention to pulmonary vascular resistance and RV dysfunction. In the second part, Dr. Mark Farber elaborates on the development of peripheral edema with special consideration of renal and hormonal abnormalities.

Finally, Dr. Anthony Cosentino provides an outstanding chapter on the therapeutic use of mechanical ventilation based on his lifetime of professional expertise and unique wisdom. This remarkable discussion includes a complete delineation of history, development, definitions, utilization, insight, experience, strategies, disease states, and weaning—all afforded by his thorough understanding of the optimal application of ventilatory support in the management of hundreds of patients with cardiopulmonary dysfunction over the past forty years.

Dean T. Mason, M.D.
Physician-in-Chief, Western Heart Institute
Chairman, Department of Cardiovascular Medicine
St. Mary's Medical Center, San Francisco
Editor-in-Chief, American Heart Journal
Past President, American College of Cardiology

Contents

Physiology:
Heart, Lungs, and Thorax

Anthony M. Cosentino, M.D.

Ode to a Fish
Hail to thee aquatic wonder
Whose gill apparatus never blunders
Gills that flutter, leave no doubt
Oxygen in, Carbon dioxide out.
Non cogitas sed es*
Simple is the best
But alas you left the brine, for the earth to feel
And now our lung is our Achilles heel.
*You do not think but you are.

Basic Physiology

As the effective gas exchange surface retreated from the ambient environment, a number of adaptations were necessary and occurred. A series of low-resistance conduits allow air to pass from mouth to alveolar gas exchange surface with a minimum of resistance. An intricate network of branching small airways in parallel minimizes resistance to flow. A much more difficult problem, however, was created by the air-liquid interface, unique to air-breathing animals. We shall see that the surface for gas exchange is potentially a very unstable surface, one that is subject to collapse and flooding and is also a source of significant resistance to expansion. The

From: Cosentino AM, Martin RJ (eds.): Cardiothoracic Interrelationships in Clinical Practice. © Futura Publishing Co., Inc., Armonk, NY, 1997.

movement of air from mouth to alveolus requires that work be done, and to accomplish this a group of specialized muscles for respiration coupled with a magnificently designed osseous structure, the rib cage, evolved. It was determined that the heart would reside within the thoracic cage. This unique living arrangement, or cohabitation, is the subject of this book.

Mechanics, Part I

Under normal conditions and at rest, airflow resistance is minimal. The pressure drop associated with laminar flow is directly proportional to $\dot{V}$.

$\Delta P \propto \dot{V}$ and the proportionality constant, K, is resistance, i.e., centimeters of water (cm H_2O) per liter per sec (L/s). Therefore,

$$\Delta P = K \dot{V} \text{ and } K = R \qquad \Delta P = R \dot{V}$$
$$R = \Delta P/\dot{V} = \text{cm } H_2O \text{ per } L/s \tag{1}$$

The pressure drop associated with turbulent flow is much greater for a given flow rate.

$$\Delta Pturb \propto V^2 \tag{2}$$

Turbulent flow occurs at each branch point in the tracheobronchial tree. However, an intricate system of peripheral branching airways functions much as a series of parallel electrical circuits, wherein resistance is inversely related to the number of parallel placed circuits.

$$1/R = 1/r + 1/r_2 + 1/r_3, \text{ etc. and } R \propto 1/n \tag{3}$$

Consequently, flow resistance in a normal individual is small and the major component is in proximal airways,[1,2] the majority in the first ten airway generations (Figure 1).

The normal flow resistance is about 1.0 cm H_2O per L/s.[3] Flow rates during normal breathing are sinusoidal and vary from 300 L/s to about 1.0 L/s, which requires a pressure gradient across the lung of about 1 cm H_2O. A narrowing of the proximal major airways, as can occur with a tumor or acute bronchial asthma, may result in a significant increase in flow resistance, which can sometimes be life threatening.

A greater resistance to air movement is encountered in the elastic structure of the lung.[3] This may be expressed as the pressure change per unit of lung expansion, i.e., cm H_2O/L and is referred to as elastance. The reciprocal of this resistance is referred to as compliance. This value is obtained by measuring inflation pressures at a series of lung volumes and at points of no air flow. A plot of P versus V, however, yields a curve that is not linear and, in fact, the deflation limb is not superimposed on the inflation curve (Figure 2). This latter phenomenon is referred to as hysteresis. The alinearity of the

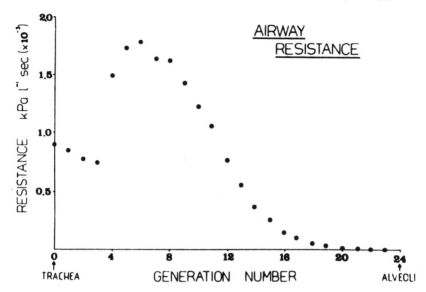

Figure 1. Resistance of each generation down the tracheo-bronchial tree from trachea (0) to smallest airways (23), calculated assuming Poiseuille flow and using the symmetrical model of Weibel (1963). (Reprinted with permission from W.B. Saunders Co., Philadelphia Scientific Foundations of Respiratory Medicine, (ed) Scadding, Cumming, Thurlbock, p., 124.)

curve may be attributed to the fact that volume is a function of radius^3, i.e., volume of a sphere $= 2/3\,\pi\,r^3$. Further compliance is of necessity related to total surface area. Pressure is force per unit area and a pressure applied to a larger surface area will produce a greater change in volume than if applied to a smaller surface. The compliance of a lung of a small animal and that of an elephant are similar. Compliance related to lung volume is referred to as specific compliance. Patients with adult respiratory distress syndrome (ARDS) are thought of as having stiff or non-compliant lungs. In fact, the apparent low compliance is better explained on the basis of only a small part of the lung seeing mouth pressure, a phenomenon worthy of consideration in understanding ventilator strategies in ARDS (see Chapter 8, Mechanical Ventilation). Finally, although we measure compliance or elastance at points of no air flow, in fact, work to overcome elastic resistance is expended continuously as the lung expands; the elastic resistance to deformation is frequency dependent, a fact that is lost if we regard elastic resistance as a resistance to be considered only at points of no airflow. The relationship of elastance and frequency is best approximated as a reactance:

$$\text{Reactance} = 1 \div 2\pi f C \quad C = \text{capacitance (compliance)} \qquad (4)$$

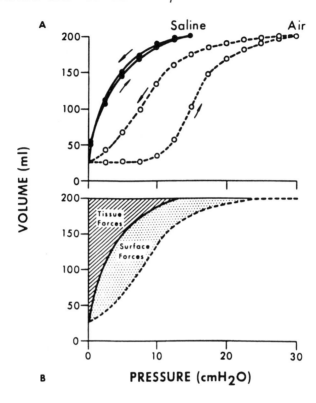

Figure 2. Effect of air-water interface of lung distensibility. Top: Note hysteresis that is lost as lungs are inflated with saline. Bottom: Relative work required to distend lung as a function of surface active force and tissue elastic forces. Dashed line represents the average of the inflation and deflation limbs of the air inflation and deflation curves. (Reprinted with permission from Clements JA, Tierney DF: Alveolar instability associated with altered surface tension. In: Fenn WO, Rahn H (eds). Handbook of Physiology, Section 3, Respiration, vol II, pp 1565–1583. Washington, DC, American Physiological Society, 1965.)

How do we relate airflow resistance and the resistance we call elastance or reactance? R is expressed as cm $H_2O/L/s$ and El as cm H_2O/L. The units are dissimilar and cannot be added algebraically. Rather, they are added geometrically so that $Z = \sqrt{R^2 + (1 \div 2\pi fC)^2}$ (Figure 3).[4]

Thus, we see that it is impedance that the respiratory pump must overcome. Furthermore, we see that conditions associated with increased elastic resistance, e.g., pulmonary fibrosis, might be expected to manifest increased respiratory frequency, f, so as to minimize work of breathing[5] as regularly observed. In subjects with increased airways resistance, work of breathing should be less at lower frequencies. Thus, it is a seeming paradox

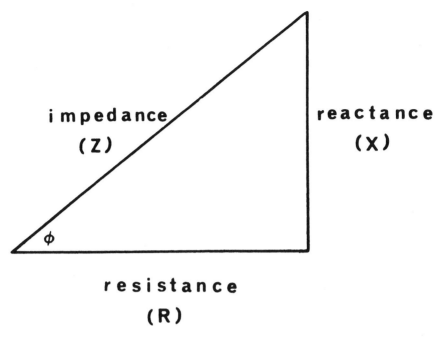

Figure 3. Although Compliance (C), the reciprocal of elastic resistance, is measured at points of no airflow, elastic resistance is continually encountered during inflation. This resistive element is best described as a reactance (X). (Note the inverse relationship to "f".) $X = 1 \div 2\pi fC$. The total impedance (Z) of a circuit, expressed in ohms is a geometrical summation of resistance (flow resistance = pressure/flow) and reactance. This geometrical relationship is expressed by the Pythagorean theorem. $Z = \sqrt{R^2 + (1 \div 2\pi fC)^2}$.

that status asthmaticus is associated with an increased respiratory rate. This will be addressed in the management of status asthmaticus.

Let us further examine the source of elastic resistance manifested by the lung. In the early 1900s, von Neergard [6] noted that a water-filled lung, i.e., one without an air-liquid interface, could be inflated with about one-quarter the distending pressure as an air-filled lung and furthermore, a liquid-filled lung did not demonstrate hysteresis (Figure 2). von Neergard[6] correctly attributed this phenomenon to surface tension, a force present at any dissimilar interface. Thus, insects can walk on water thanks to the elastic film at the air-liquid interface. Pattle[7] reasoned that this force could create a tremendous collapsing tendency and that a surface-active detergent was necessary to maintain a low enough surface tension to prevent alveolar collapse, i.e., alveolar instability. Note that this collapsing tendency also results in a pressure gradient from alveolar capillary to alveolus that favors the formation of alveolar flooding[8] and thus "surfactant" both stabilizes alveolar volume and discourages the formation of pulmonary edema. Brown[9] subsequently isolated and characterized this material as dipalmitoylphosphatidyl choline. Its action in life is probably facilitated by the presence of unsaturated or negatively charged phospholipids plus an azoprotein. This topic has been reviewed by Goerke and Clements.[10]

Mechanics, Part II

Air flows from mouth to alveolus as a result of positive pressure gradient whether spontaneous or mechanically assisted. Mouth pressure of sea level during spontaneous ventilation is 1000 cm H_2O, 760 mm Hg or 32 ft H_2O. Air flow occurs because pleural pressure and alveolar pressure becomes subatmospheric as a result of the contraction of the respiratory muscles coupled with a "stable" chest wall that resists inward deformation. The principal muscle responsible for generating this pressure gradient or transpulmonary pressure is the diaphragm, an organ once thought to be the seat of the soul (phrene indicates soul, mind, schizophrenia indicates split soul). During normal inspiration then pleural pressure (Ppl) becomes subatmospheric, and in the presence of a severe mechanical load, Ppl may reach levels in excess of 50 cm H_2O subatmospheric. Exhalation is essentially passive and results from elastic recoil generated during inspiration. At end expiration in normal subjects the interplay of the elastic properties of the chest wall and of the lungs results in a Ppl (pleural pressure) of about −5 cm H_2O, i.e., 5 cm H_2O subatmospheric. Because this pressure is related to lung volume and the compliance of the chest wall, diseases associated with hyperinflation result in a less subatmospheric pressure and those associated with small lung volumes represent a greater (more negative) subatmospheric pressure. This phenomenon is to be reckoned with in understanding blood flow into and out of the thorax and in the interpretation of the jugular venous pulse.

Pulmonary Blood Flow

The pressure in the pulmonary circulation is relatively low, approximately 25/10 with a mean of 15 mm Hg in the pulmonary artery. Since the adult upright lung is about 30 cm high, hydrostatic pressures play a significant role in pulmonary blood flow, i.e., the lung bases will have a significantly higher perfusing pressure than the lung apices, 30 cm H_2O or 23 mm Hg. Furthermore, the pulmonary capillaries are exposed to alveolar air that is significantly different than Ppl. Figure 4 is a tracing from a wedged pulmonary artery catheter. Note the marked respiratory fluctuations. To obviate the effects of the respiratory fluctuations, the wedge pres-

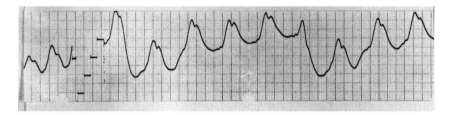

Figure 4. A tracing from a "wedged" pulmonary artery catheter. Patient is breathing spontaneously. Note respiratory fluctuations. PA occlusion pressure should be measured at end expiration. Electronic averaging may seriously underestimate Ppao.

sure is measured at end expiration, a point at which alveolar pressure approximates atmospheric pressure.

In clinical practice this single value represents the filling pressure of the heart and also capillary pressure that tends to drive fluid out of the pulmonary capillaries. We shall see in the discussion of cardiac performance that this is a gross oversimplification.

Measurements of pulmonary blood flow have resulted in some fascinating observations. Blood flow in most vascular beds is proportional to the difference between arterial and venous pressure. Permutt[11] and Permutt and Riley[12] observed, however, that in the lung there is a zone where raising venous pressure up to a point produces no change in pulmonary blood flow, or conversely, lowering venous pressure below that point failed to augment flow (Figure 5).

Permutt[11] "reasoned that this was due to a zone in which alveolar pressure exceeded venous pressure and flow behaved as if passing through a waterfall. This can be simulated in the laboratory with a Starling resistor, a semicollapsible tube (Figure 6).

In this figure, Pa > Pa|v > Pv and blood flow is α to Pa − Pa|v. This is referred to as zone II in the lung. In zone I, Pa|v > Pa > Pv and theoretically there is no blood flow to this zone. This situation probably does not exist in normal individuals but may exist if PA pressure is abnormally low or Pa|v is abnormally elevated, e.g., mechanical ventilation and/or auto-positive end-expiratory pressure (auto-PEEP), i.e., Pa|v is supra-atmospheric at end expiration. In zone III Pa > Pa|v < Pv and blood flow is proportional to Pa − Pv.

In zone IV, blood flow curiously is noted to decrease (Figure 7).[13] It is postulated that the major resistance to flow shifts to extra-alveolar vessels, which are subject to increases in interstitial pressures such as in pulmonary edema. Vascular tone, however, may also play a role.

Pulmonary blood flow exhibits other anomalous behavior that makes the calculation of pulmonary vascular resistance problematic. Classically, resistance (Flow ÷ (Pa − Pv) should remain constant over a range of blood flows. Furthermore, this is a first-order equation, which says flow should be

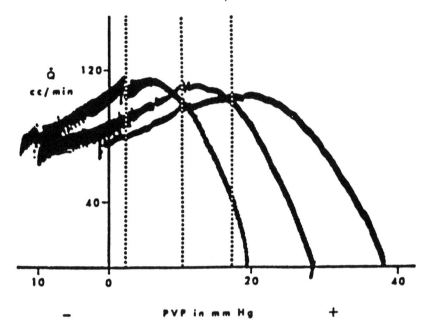

Figure 5. The relationship between flow (Q̇ and pulmonary venous pressure (PVP) at three different pulmonary arterial pressures and alveolar pressures in the left lower lobe of an open chest dog. As venous pressure decreases (going from right to left) flow increases to the point where venous pressure equals alveolar pressure. At that point, a further decrease in venous pressure fails to increase flow (zone II). The relationship between flow (Q̇) and pulmonary venous pressure (PVP) at three different pulmonary arterial pressures and alveolar pressures in the left lower lobe of an open chest dog. (Reproduced with permission from Medicina Thoracalis. Permutt S, et al. Alveolar pressure pulmonary venous pressure and the vascular waterfall. Medic Thorac 1962;19:245.)

linear and the curve should pass through the origin; this in fact is not true. The curve is not linear and does not pass through the origin (Figure 8).[14]

The slope of this line should be resistance, but we see that the slope is not constant and, in fact, resistance appears to decrease as flow increases. The issue is whether to calculate pulmonary vascular resistance (PVR) as the slope of the line over the linear portion of the curve or as two separate curves with both lines passing through zero, as is customarily done. This latter strategy leads the clinician to conclude that PVR decreases as flow increases. An alternative is that the early portion of the curve reflects a pressure drop required for pulmonary vascular recruitment and that PVR is more appropriately calculated as the slope of the rectilinear portion of the curve. Clearly right ventricular (RV) work in the normal person is minimal and increased flow, as occurs during exercise may occur with little change in pressure.

STARLING RESISTOR

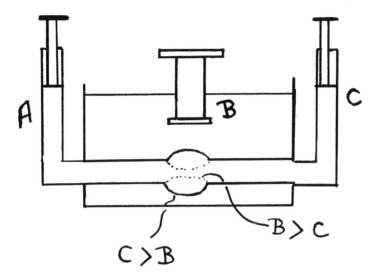

Figure 6. A model of the lung analogous to a Starling resistor.

A further confounding factor about PVR might be expected to occur with tidal breathing and with changes in lung volumes as occurs in disease states. The data and conclusions that relate to this topic have generated great controversy. A major area of disagreement among investigators has concerned the seemingly different effects of negative pressure versus positive pressure inflation on pulmonary mechanics.[15-17] It has been suggested that positive pressure ventilation increases PVR and that negative pressure ventilation does not, and may, in fact, decrease PVR.[18] The explanation for this apparent difference becomes apparent when the experimental models are examined. In the studies of Burton and Patel,[16] and those of Thomas et al.,[15] inflation of the lung was accomplished by reduction of pressure in a chamber surrounding the lung. The airway and blood perfusion systems were kept at atmospheric pressure. A decrease in box pressure produced an increase in transmural pressure of the larger pulmonary vessels and thus, lowered the resistance of the system. For any degree of lung inflation, whether produced by negative pressure or positive pressure, the transpulmonary pressure, and thus, "the tension on the lung wall is the same" (Vischer, Rupp, and Scott[19]). There is no reason why the effect on the capillaries in the lung wall should be different. Whittenberger[17] concluded that a highly distended lung has a

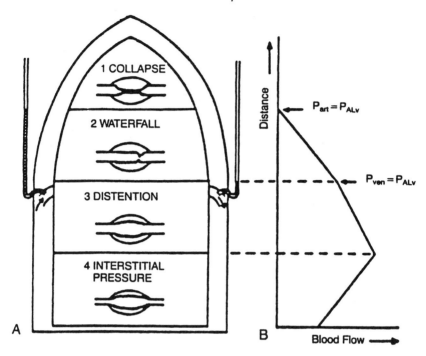

Figure 7. Regional distribution of pulmonary blood flow. (A) A diagram that shows the factors affecting blood flow in zones 1,2,3, and 4. (B) A diagram that shows regional blood flow per unit of lung volume at corresponding levels within the lung. (From Hughes JMB, Glazier JB, Maloney JE, et al: Effect of lung volume on the distribution of pulmonary blood flow in man. Respir Physiol 4:58–72, 1968. With permission.)

high vascular resistance. He further concluded these findings were not due to changes of lung volume per se, but rather were more closely associated with changes in tranpulmonary pressure. He reasoned that with creation of a transpulmonary pressure associated with lung inflation, there must exist a pressure gradient across lung tissue that increases the pressure to which blood vessels are exposed and those closest to alveoli should be affected most. The extrapulmonary vessels that are exposed to Ppl should be least affected. Furthermore, the level at which transpulmonary pressure increased PVR was inversely related to pulmonary artery pressure.

In summary, increases in tidal volume during exercise result in only minimal changes in pressure with significant increases in cardiac output. Experimentally high degrees of lung inflation, whether produced by negative or positive pressure breathing may result in an increase in PVR. This is believed to be a consequence of an increase in transpulmonary pressure that affects predominantly the pulmonary capillaries.

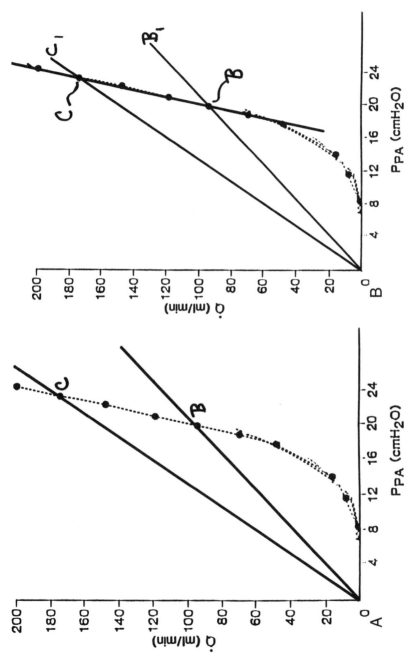

Figure 8. Blood flow versus PPA. If we assume pulmonary artery flow versus pressure is linear and passes through zero, it appears that resistance decreases as flow increases. In fact, flow versus pressure is not linear initially and does not pass through zero. However, there is a segment where the slope, i.e. resistance, is linear. Clearly BC is a very different slope than AB or AC. (Reproduced with permission from Graham, et al. J Appl Physiol, 1968, p. 1278.)

The effects of exercise or pulmonary artery pressure and PVR in disease states will be examined in the chapter on cor pulmonale.

Circulation

We shall see that there are striking similarities between ventilatory and cardiac performance. These similarities are linked with the cohabitation of the lungs and heart in a common chamber: the thorax.

Air flows into the lungs because the ventilatory pump creates a pressure difference from mouth to alveolus. Blood flows out of the chest because the cardiac pump creates a pressure difference between the thorax and systemic circulation. Air leaves the lungs as a result of elastic recoil, and in fact, elastic recoil is a major determinant of maximum expiratory flow. The reader is referred to the classic work of Hyatt and Wilcox[20] who demonstrated that maximum expiratory flow is a function of lung volume and elastic recoil and independent of expiratory effort (Figure 9).

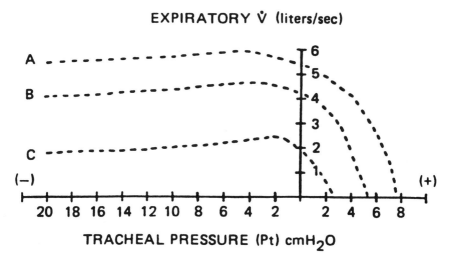

Figure 9. Effect of lung volume on isovolumic pressure-flow curves. Note that maximum flow is independent of expiratory effort; it is a function of lung volume and elastic recoil pressure. Note the similarity to cardiac venous return curves and also pulmonary blood flow in Zone II. Attention was called to this striking similarity by Permutt, Wise and Sylvester. (Reproduced with permission from Marcel Dekker, Inc. New York. Circulatory and Ventilatory Pump Interaction in the Thorax. Roussos and Macklem (eds), p. 703.)

Venous Return

Similarly, blood flow returns to the heart as a result of the elastic recoil of the systemic blood vessels and the volume of blood in the circulation. Right atrial (RA) pressure figures into the equation only if it is greater than atmospheric pressure under which conditions venous return is proportional to the recoil pressure of the systemic vessels minus RA pressure. However, at the point that RA pressure becomes subatmospheric, venous return becomes maximum, i.e., a further decrease in RA pressure relative to atmospheric pressure does not augment venous return.[21] This behavior suggests a flow-limiting segment outside of the thorax (Figure 10) analogous to what has been described in the pulmonary circulation in zone II where Pa|v exceed PV. The situation is also reminiscent of expiratory air flow from the lung wherein maximum air flow is dependent only on lung elastic recoil and lung volume and independent of muscular effort.[20]

The cardiac output in normal persons is related lock-step to oxygen consumption.[22] The mixed venous oxygen saturation is defended at 75% or PVO$_2$ of 40 mm Hg. Anemia is normally compensated for by an increase in cardiac output.

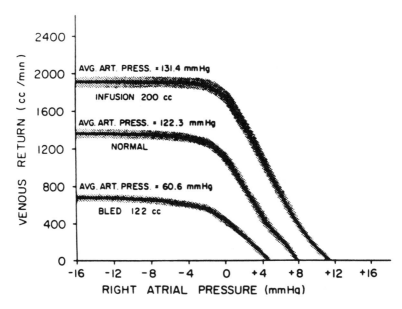

Figure 10. Venous return curves. Note that below a certain level of atrial pressure a further decline in atrial pressure fails to augment venous return. These studies were performed in the open chest animal and thus right atrial pressure is effectively RA transmural pressure. (Reproduced with permission from Marcel Dekker. Circulatory and Ventilatory Pump Interaction in the Thorax. Roussos and Macklem (eds), p. 703.)

Cardiac Performance

Frank and Starling[23] in their classic experiment demonstrated that cardiac output (CO) was a function of end-diastolic fiber length only to a point, beyond which CO was observed to decline. Some medical students are still taught that there is a descending limb of Starling's curve.[24] However, it should be noted that the relationship of filling pressure to left ventricular end-diastolic volume (LVEDV) is not so simple and may vary depending upon the mechanical properties of the ventricle (Figure 11).

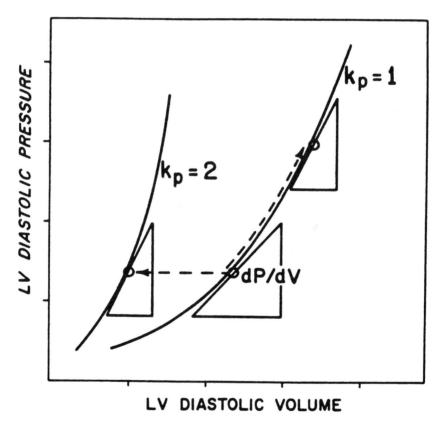

Figure 11. Diagrammatic representation of left ventricular (LV) diastolic pressure-volume relationships. Right, An increase in operative chamber stiffness (dP/dV) occurs in the absence of any change in the modulus of chamber stiffness (K_p). Left, An increase in operative chamber stiffness occurs as a result of an increase in the modulus of chamber stiffness (relative to the curve on the right). Because operative chamber stiffness depends on the modulus of stiffness and the level of operative filling pressure, this comparison is made at equivalent levels of pressure. (From Gaasch, W. H., et al.: Left ventricular compliance: mechanisms and clinical implications. Am. J. Cardiol. 38:645, 1976.)

In recent years, Starling's curve has been interpreted by Sarnoff et al.[25] as a series of ventricular function curves (Figure 12).

It is reasoned that because of the laborious procedures required to measure CO in 1918, it was late in the experiment when CO was measured at higher LVEDVs and that the descending limb observed was a reflection of depressed myocardial contractility that resulted from prolonged anesthesia and that, in fact, the animal's heart was functioning on a depressed curve. Frank and Starling[23] lacked an electromagnetic flow meter, which was available to Sarnoff, to measure CO instantaneously and repeatedly as filling pressure was varied. However, Sarnoff performed his studies in open chest animals, and thus filling pressure was LVEDP minus atmospheric pressure. The situation in the closed chest is more complex. Take a carton of milk from sea level to altitude and the carton will bulge. The filling or distending pressure is the intraluminal pressure minus the atmospheric pressure, i.e., the transmural pressure. The filling pressure of the heart is the atrial pressure minus the pericardial pressure, which under most circumstances, can be equated with pleural pressure. The latter can be approximated by measures of esophageal pressure. Note that the effective filling pressure is the determinant of fiber length.

Preload is often thought of as the ventricular end-diastolic fiber length or ventricular end-diastolic volume. It is often used interchangeably with end-diastolic pressure, and in the absence of mitral stenosis, is equated with the pulmonary capillary wedge pressure. In fact, preload is more accurately defined as atrial pressure minus pleural pressure, a relationship unfortunately

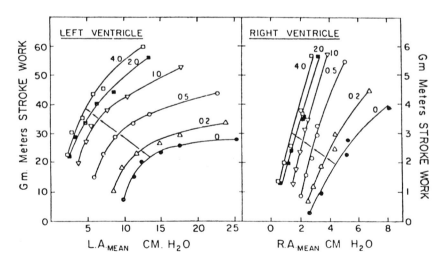

Figure 12. Filling pressures versus stroke work. This figure demonstrates the recent interpretation of the Frank-Starling mechanism. Note the absence of a descending limb. (Reproduced with permission from Sarnoff SJ. Physiol Rev 35:107–122, 1955.)

often overlooked except in cases of pericardial tamponade at which time preload or transmural pressure is decreased in spite of an elevated atrial pressure.

Afterload can be defined as systolic wall tension at the onset of ventricular ejection. It is often equated with mean aortic root pressure, a misleading oversimplification. Again, it is transmural pressure that is of interest or Pao minus Ppl. Intrapleural pressures associated with upper airways obstruction or during an acute asthmatic episode may be 50–100 cm H_2O subatmospheric. In addition, wall tension is a function of radius, i.e., $T = Pr \div 2h$; h refers to wall thickness. Pulmonary edema associated with upper airways obstruction is well documented. The relationship of obstructive sleep apnea to left ventricular disease is of interest, but remains to be documented.[26] The effects of negative intrapleural pressures during status asthmaticus will also be influenced by the marked changes in lung volumes.[27] Thus, it should be apparent that changes in Ppl can markedly influence preload and afterload with significant effect on cardiac performance.

Myocardial Contractility. We have seen that for any given filling pressure, cardiac output may vary depending upon the contractile state of the

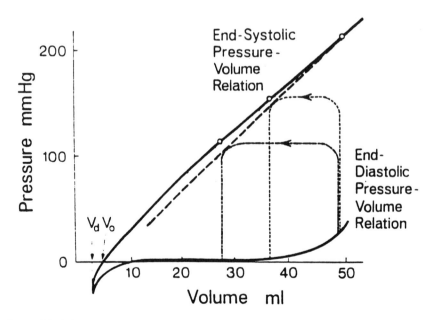

Figure 13. Schematic diagram for end-systolic pressure-volume relation and its parameters V_o and V_d. Three open circles on the solid line represent three isovolumic peak pressures. The broken line represents the end-systolic pressure-volume relation line obtained from two ejecting contraction loops as opposed to the isovolumic pressure-volume relation line. (Reproduced with permission from Sagawa K. The end-systolic pressure–volume relation of the ventricle. Circulation 63:1223–1227;1981.)

myocardium. Historically, many parameters have been examined to evaluate the functional state of the myocardium.

1. Change in volume per unit of time, i.e., dV ÷ dt.
2. Change in pressure per unit of time, i.e., dP ÷ dt.
3. Ejection fraction.
4. CO versus filling pressure.

All of the above suffer a major limitation. They fail to consider preload and/or afterload. If preload is increased, the ventricle may respond with an increase in dP ÷ dt solely due to an increase in preload and no change in contractility. One may correct for this by relating dP ÷ dt to filling pressure, i.e., dP ÷ dt ÷ P.

Similarly, CO versus filling pressure may fail to consider afterload. A classic example of this is right ventricular (RV) performance in cor pulmonale (see Chapter 7, Cor Pulmonale). If we plot CO or stroke index (SI)

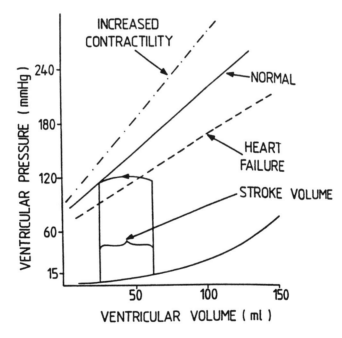

Figure 14. A diagrammatic representation of the relation between left ventricular volume and pressure. The end-systolic pressure volume relation is linear, but it is displaced downward and to the right in heart failure and upwards and to the left when contractility is increased. An idealized pressure/volume loop is included (arrow), and the curvilinear line represents the end-diastolic pressure/volume relation. (Reproduced with permission from MacNee W. Pathophysiology of Cor Pulmonale in COPD. Am J Respir Crit Care Med 150:833–852;1994.)

versus right ventricular end-diastolic pressure (RVEDP), the curve is flat and appears to be abnormal, but normalizes when we plot stroke work index (SWI) versus RVEDP.[28]

Clearly, a true measure of myocardial contractility should be independent of preload and/or afterload. This dilemma was defined by Sagawa and colleagues[29] in the 1970s, when they proposed that myocardial contractility could be assessed by examining the end-systolic pressure-volume ratio. They showed in an experimental model and subsequently in the human left ventricle that this simple relation was independent of pre- and afterloading conditions. Furthermore, three laboratories[30-32] reported a linear relationship between end-systolic pressure and volume in the physiological range, and in many studies was shown to separate normal from poorly contracting left ventricles. MacNee[33] has subsequently shown that this relationship can be used to assess the contractility of the right ventricle (Figures 13 and 14).

Summary

Venous return is a function of blood volume and the elastic recoil of the capacitance vessels of the peripheral circulation. RA pressure influences venous return only if pressure is greater than atmospheric pressure. Further decreases in RA pressure do not augment venous return.

Blood flow through the pulmonary circulation is accomplished with little force required by the right ventricle once pulmonary capillaries have been recruited. Alveolar pressure, when greater than pulmonary venous pressure, can profoundly affect regional blood flow. Degree of lung inflation may significantly affect pulmonary vascular resistance (see Chapter 7, Cor Pulmonale).

Cardiac output in the normal resting and exercising person responds in a lock-step fashion to oxygen consumption so that mixed venous oxygen content is rigidly regulated to be 75% saturated or a PaO_2 of about 40 mm Hg. Cardiac output responds to changes in filling pressures in compliance with the Frank-Starling law of the heart. However, this law is best expressed as a series of ventricular function curves that vary with changes in myocardial contractility. The filling pressures or preload in the absence of tricuspid or mitral stenosis is the atrial pressure minus pleural pressure. Changes in lung volume may cause changes in pleural pressure, and thus influence preload. Afterload is a function of radius of the ventricle, wall thickness, and aortic root pressure minus pleural pressure. Thus, perturbations in lung mechanics can profoundly influence cardiac performance. Evaluation of the myocardial contractile state at the patient's bedside can be difficult.

Applied Physiology

In subsequent chapters, the unique relationships of heart, lung, and thorax will be explored in detail in several disease states. Several clinical dilemmas that do not justify a complete chapter are, however, worthy of discussion because they demonstrate the unique interrelationships between thoracic mechanics and cardiac performance.

Assessment of Cardiac Filling Pressure During Continuous Positive Pressure Ventilation with and without PEEP

It is recognized that changes in intrathoracic pressure during ventilation, whether spontaneous or mechanical, is associated with significant respiratory fluctuations in pressure tracings obtained from a pulmonary artery catheter. It is generally agreed that there is good correlation between the pulmonary artery occlusion pressure and the left atrial pressure even during mechanical ventilation.[34] It is conventional to measure the wedge pressure (Ppao) at end expiration, a point at which alveolar pressure is presumed to be atmospheric. The situation is less clear upon the addition of PEEP and is a topic of continuing debate.[35,36] Geer[35] and Downs and Douglas[36] called attention to this dilemma. The latter demonstrated that the addition of PEEP resulted in an increase in pressure right atrium (PRA) and Ppao, but a decrease in LV filling pressure if LV filling pressure was defined as LVEDP minus Ppl.[36] They concluded that measurement of Ppl was necessary to accurately assess LV filling pressure during continuous positive pressure ventilation (CPPV). The effects of PEEP on Ppl were unpredictable, but they cautioned against removal of PEEP to measure wedge pressure because in their experimental model, this resulted in alveolar flooding.

Smiseth et al.[37] suggested that changes in PRA accurately reflected changes in pericardial pressure (ΔPP) and thus changes in effective LV filling pressures might be more accurately assessed by subtracting the change in PRA from the observed new value of LVEDP after a particular therapeutic intervention. Thus, it may be reasoned that changes in Ppao after the addition of PEEP might be corrected for by subtracting the rise in PRA from the new value for Ppao.

Pinsky and colleagues[38] based on their studies in stable postoperative cardiac surgery patients, suggested that the addition of 5 cm H_2O PEEP produced no significant changes in Ppao, but higher levels of PEEP, 5 to 15 cm H_2O were associated with an increase in wedge pressure. Furthermore, they noted no deleterious effects in this patient population when PEEP was discontinued for

15 seconds to permit a more accurate measure of Ppao. They believed their data refuted the results of Smiseth et al.[37] Butler and Albert[39] subsequently pointed out that Pinsky misinterpreted Smiseth's conclusions and erroneously examined the absolute value of PRA rather than the change in PRA in correcting for changes in Ppao with the application of PEEP.

Furthermore, it is apparent that to understand the significance of changes in Ppao associated with addition of PEEP, knowledge of the intrapericardial pressure is required so that we may calculate transmural pressures. Marini et al.[40] demonstrated in a canine model that PEEP was associated with a lifting of the heart. This resulted in a hydrostatic increase in pressures recorded from catheters in the left atrium and mediastinum and a decrease in measurements made from an esophageal balloon as the heart was lifted from the esophagus. This helps to explain some of the discrepancies reported in studies of LV performance associated with PEEP, which will be discussed shortly. However, it also emphasizes the difficulties in the clinical interpretation of data obtained from a pulmonary artery catheter during application of PEEP.

It would appear 5 cm H_2O PEEP has little effect on the estimates of LV filling pressure as conventionally evaluated with a pulmonary artery catheter. When higher levels of PEEP are required in unstable patients, it would appear prudent not to discontinue the PEEP to evaluate LV filling pressure. Changes in PRA might be useful, as demonstrated by Smiseth.[37] However, changes in Ppao after volume infusion or diuresis rather than absolute values of Ppao might be a more practical clinical approach to this commonly encountered clinical dilemma. If a diuretic results in an increase in urine output, but no change in blood pressure or filling pressure, continue diuresis. If fluid infusion causes an abrupt increase in filling pressure, withhold fluids.

PEEP: Effects on Cardiac Output and Lung Water

It is a common observation that the addition of PEEP to a mechanically ventilated patient may be associated with a decrease in blood pressure and cardiac output.[41] Paradoxically, in patients with congestive heart failure (CHF) PEEP may be associated with an increase in cardiac performance manifested as an increase in cardiac output and decrease in LV filling pressure.[42]

The observed effects of PEEP in subjects with normal LV function have been attributed to a decrease in venous return secondary to an increase in RA pressure. Furthermore, it has been proposed that increases in lung volume may increase PVR and RV afterload with a resultant leftward shift of the interventricular septum.[34] Other studies have suggested diminished LV contractility.[43]

Jardin et al.[34] using a single view two-dimensional echocardiography technique purported to show that there was a leftward septal shift associated with a decrease in LV end-diastolic transmural pressure and thus concluded that the principle effect of PEEP was an increase in PVR and RV afterload with an enlarged RV that limited LV filling as a result of ventricular interdependence. Animal studies have reported PEEP-related increases in LV transmural pressure and have suggested LV dysfunction.[43] We have seen earlier, however, that the measurements of LV transmural pressure are fraught with difficulties and that more accurate measurements of pericardial pressure have failed to substantiate these findings. Further, the studies of Jardin[34] used levels of PEEP as great as 30 cm H_2O.

Three subsequent studies that used lower levels of PEEP are in agreement.[44–46] Viquerat[44] used equilibrium radionuclide angiography and concluded the primary mechanism was a decrease in venous return. Terai et al.[45] used transesophageal echocardiography and noted that RA and RVEDV volume decreased immediately when PEEP was applied and left atrial end-diastolic dimensions began to decrease a few seconds later. They concluded LV preload decreased as a result of a decrease in RV preload and thus CO was reduced as a result of the decrease in RV and LV preload. Potkin et al.[46] also used equilibrium radionuclide angiography and concluded that the major effect of PEEP is a reduction in preload of both ventricles. RV and LV ejection fractions did not decline with increasing levels of PEEP. There was no evidence for depressed LV function.

Thus, it would appear the dilemma is solved. However, controversy persists over the mechanism for the decrease in venous return and a unifying concept that might explain the improvement in cardiac performance when PEEP is added to subjects with LV dysfunction.

Certainly PEEP increases PPI PRA relative to the atmospheric pressure. However, the pressure gradient for venous return is the pressure in the systemic capacitance vessels, PMS minus PRA until PRA becomes subatmospheric. Mean systemic pressure, PMS, is related to the elastic recoil of the systemic capacitance vessels and the blood volume. Curiously, the application of PEEP has not been associated with a decrease in the pressure gradient, i.e., PMS increased an amount equal to the rise in PRA.[47]

One is inclined to attribute this observation to a rise in intra-abdominal pressure. However, a significant role for abdominal pressure could not be demonstrated in this study, nor in the study of Scharf et al.[48] who found equal decreases in CO with PEEP with the abdomen intact, open, or bound. However, after carotid sinus and vagal denervation or total spinal anesthesia, the increase in PMS was significantly mitigated.[48] Permutt concluded that the increase in PMS, associated with PEEP was due both to reflex and mechanical factors and that under control conditions, PEEP does not decrease the difference between PMS and PRA. A third mechanism that may increase PMS during PEEP is the translocation of blood from the central to the systemic circulation and thus support cardiac output.[49] This may explain the observation that in CHF, PEEP may result in decreased congestive phenomena. It would appear reasonable to speculate that there might be a greater redistribution of blood from the congested central circulation, i.e., lungs and heart, to the periphery. Also, because CHF is associated with an increase in PVR, the systemic circulation might be expected to be less compliant, and thus, an even greater rise in PMS could result. A condition such as cor pulmonale that is not associated with an increase in PVR or an increase in central blood volume would predictably result in a profound decrease in cardiac output and blood pressure.

The observation remains, however, that PEEP does result in a decrease in venous return. If the pressure gradient for venous return is not diminished, it follows that there must be an increase in vascular resistance somewhere between the capacitance vessels and the thorax or that, in fact there is a flow limiting segment comparable to zone II in the pulmonary circulation where alveolar pressure becomes the limiting pressure. Experimental data in the dog submitted by Fessler and colleagues,[50] in fact, supports this theory. The reader is referred to the discussion of this topic by Fessler and Permutt.[51]

In summary, PEEP results in a decrease in venous return. The mechanism remains controversial but may be associated with flow-limiting segment outside of the thorax. Preload is decreased in both the right and left ventricle. Increase in RV afterload has been reported with very high levels of PEEP, but not confirmed. Documentation of LV dysfunction is lacking. PEEP often results in clinical improvement in CHF by displacing blood from the thorax to the periphery. An increase in intrapleural pressure may decrease LV afterload and thus increase cardiac output.

PEEP and Pulmonary Edema

It was first demonstrated in 1909 that application of positive airway pressure was beneficial in experimental pulmonary edema.[52] It is agreed that CPPV is also beneficial in pulmonary edema associated with LV failure, but the mechanism remains unclear. At first it would seem to be due to positive pressure pushing fluid from the alveoli as proposed by Emerson[52] and by Barach et al.[53] However, an increase in mouth pressure is associated with an increase in all intrathoracic pressures including vascular pressures so that there is no net increase in pressure gradient from alveolus to capillary. As previously noted, there will be changes in vascular pressure gradients from thoracic to systemic vessels, which may influence central blood volume as a result of effects on both preload and afterload. However, if PEEP does have an effect on the formation and/or clearance of pulmonary edema independent of effects on cardiac function, it must, of necessity, be secondary to changes in transpulmonary pressure that equates with an increase in lung volume. It follows that if increased lung volume causes a change in lung water, it should make no difference whether the increase in transpulmonary pressure and lung volume occurs as a result of spontaneous breathing or supra-atmospheric mouth pressure. The effects of PEEP on fluid formation and/or clearance remains unclear. The major therapeutic effect in pulmonary edema, upon which there is agreement, is that it increases the ratio of air to liquid in flooded alveoli.[54] Further, in CHF, it has been reported to be associated with an increase in cardiac output.[55] These observations will be reexamined in formulating a ventilator support strategy for patients with altered cardiac function (see Chapter 8, Mechanical Ventilation).

Pulsus Paradoxus and Bronchial Asthma

Pulsus paradoxus is defined as an exaggerated decline in systolic arterial pressure during inspiration, usually of a magnitude > 10 mm Hg. Kussmaul[56] observed and reported this phenomena in 1873 and associated his observations with constrictive pericarditis. It is now recognized that pulsus paradoxus is infrequently seen with constrictive pericarditis, but is a valuable sign of pericardial tamponade.[57] It may also be seen in severe CHF, severe asthma, and tension pneumothorax. The mechanism is controversial, but several theories have been proposed.[58]

1. Pooling of blood in the lungs.
2. Increase in LV afterload associated with a decrease in PPI.
3. Deviation of the interventricular septum during inspiration with a resultant increase in RV volume and decrease in LV volume.
4. Decrease in LV filling due to a decrease in RV output secondary to increase lung volume and an increase in pulmonary vascular resistance.

Because pulsus paradoxus is an exaggerated response to inspiration it is appropriate to examine the usual effects of respiration on cardiac performance. Robotham et al.[59] reported an increase in LV filling pressures associated with inspiratory efforts with both constant and increasing lung volume in anesthetized dogs. They concluded that the decrease in LV stroke volume was due to an increase in LV afterload. In a subsequent study that used spontaneously breathing dogs on right heart bypass, the effect of the Muller maneuver was studied.[60] Again, they noted a decrease in LV stroke volume and an increase in LV transmural pressure and afterload. However, when the right heart was allowed to fill and right heart volume increased, the decline in LV stroke volume was significantly greater. They concluded that the decrease in LV stroke volume was due to both an increase in LV afterload associated with a decrease in PPI and also to an increase in right heart volume.

Scharf et al.[61] studied anesthetized dogs during quiet respiration and breathing with inspiratory loading before and after vagotomy intended to prolong inspiration. They achieved results similar to those of Robotham and reached similar conclusions.[62]

Guz, Innes, and Murphy[63] documented with pulsed Doppler ultrasound that LV stroke volume did fall during inspiration and that the changes in stroke volume varied directly with increasing tidal volume. Breath holding abolished the variance in stroke volume. However, an increase in respiratory resistance also accentuated the inspiratory decline in LV stroke volume and, in fact, total occlusion of the airway that prevented a change in lung volume was still accompanied by a decrease in LV stroke volume associated with the effort at inspiration. However, the magnitude of changes was not large in spite of large fluctuations in intrathoracic pressures. Curiously, when the studies were repeated in subjects who had undergone a pericardiectomy, the respiratory changes in LV stroke volume were significantly decreased, but not abolished. This study suggests that paradoxical pulse is in part, related to an inspiratory shift of the interventricular septum from right to left with a decrease in LV volume and may in part be related to an increase in LV afterload due to a decrease in PPI with a resultant increase in LV transmural pressure.

Sometimes forgotten is that pulsus paradoxus was first described in 1717 in association with attacks of bronchial asthma.[64] Unique to the asthmatic state is an increase in airways resistance, markedly negative intrapleural pressures during inspiration, a modest increase in expiratory pleural pressures, hyperinflation, and a tendency for alveolar pressure to remain supra-atmospheric at end expiration,[65] a phenomenon referred to as auto-PEEP. In the report of Jardin et al.[66] hemodynamic studies, echocardiography, and esophageal pressures were recorded in nine subjects with status asthmaticus. Esophageal pressures varied from about -25 cm H_2O in inspiration to about 8 cm H_2O in expiration.

There was a leftward shift of the intraventricular septum associated with an increase in RV dimensions and decrease in LV dimensions. At first glance, it might appear that there is a large increase in venous return to the right ventricle during inspiration, that results in RV dilatations, septal displacement, and decrease in LV dimensions in spite of an increase in LV transmural pressure, i.e., LVEDP minus PPI. However, the studies of Guyton demonstrate that there is a maximum effect of lowering right atrial pressure on venous return and further the right atrial, RV and pulmonary vasculature is a high-capacitance system. Consistent with this information is that in this study of Jardin,[66] the initial part of the abdominal vena cava was noted to collapse at end of inspiration, thus creating a flow-limiting segment similar to a vascular waterfall as discussed earlier in this chapter. Why then, the increase in RV volume during inspiration? Jardin and colleagues[66] noted a decrease in pulmonary pulse pressure that was in phase with the decrease in systemic pulse pressure, i.e., both minimal during inspiration and maximal during expiration. This is contrary to the findings in cardiac tamponade where RV and LV pulse pressures have been shown to be approximately 180° out of phase.[67] They concluded that pulsus paradoxus in status asthmaticus, unlike cardiac tamponade, is not only caused by competition of RV and LV for intrapericardial space, but in addition, must include increased impedance to RV ejection.

These findings are consistent with the observations of Permutt[65] in an asthmatic subject in whom the increase in PA pressure was shown to rise lock-step with the increase in negativity of the pleural pressure. It is concluded that "RV overloading is a major hemodynamic consequence induced by markedly negative intrathoracic pressures during inspiration" (Figure 15).

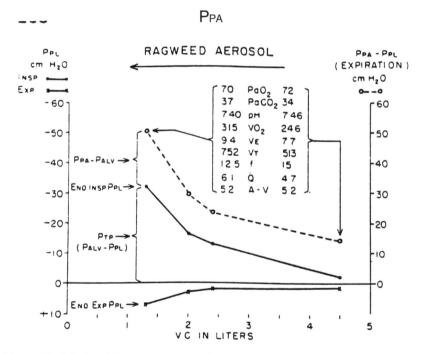

Figure 15. Relationships between pleural pressure (P_{pi}), pulmonary arterial pressure (P_{pa}), and vital capacity (VC) during the production of an acute asthmatic attack with a ragweed aerosol. The pleural pressures are treated as end-expiratory pressures for the purpose of analysis, although they are actually peak pressures. For the vertical distance between the two upper curves to represent the difference between pulmonary arterial pressure and alveolar pressure (PALV), it is necessary to assume that the static transpulmonary pressure (PTP) did not change significantly between inspiration and expiration. The numbers within brackets are measurements made before and at height of asthmatic attack. Note that the PPA, i.e. PPA—expiratory PPI, rises lock step with the progressive negativity of the inspiratory pleural pressure. (Reproduced with permission from Permutt S. Chest 63:28S:1973.)

Lung Disease and Cardiac Output

Recent studies in the laboratories of Celli[68] suggest that exercise limitation in chronic obstructive pulmonary disease (COPD) is related both to decreased cardiac performance as well as abnormal lung mechanics. Oxygen pulse,[69] a surrogate for stroke volume, failed to increase appropriately during exercise. The late Dr. Butler's group[70] demonstrated that the elevated wedge pressure observed in COPD during exercise could be reproduced simply by an equal degree of hyperpnea without exercise and concluded this was an effect of hyperinflation (auto-PEEP).

The following subject (Figure 16) with acute interstitial lung disease due to avian antigen pneumonitis, which is a small lung volume disorder, also demonstrated a profound depression of cardiac performance.[71] In

Male, age 18, high school athlete. Weight 72 kg; Height 175 cm.
Recurrent episodes of dyspnea, "pneumonitis," and radiologic diffuse pulmonary infiltration.
Diagnosis: Allergic alveolitis (bird antigen)
Treatment: Removal of antigen associated with reversal of symptoms and x-ray changes.

	March	*December*	*Predicted*
Pulmonary Function at Rest:			
Total lung capacity (l)	4.6	5.9	7.0
Vital capacity (l)	3.4	4.5	5.2
FEV_1 (l)	3.0	3.9	4.2
Diffusing capacity (CO) (ml/min/mm Hg)	14	24	30
Exercise Studies:			
1. Maximal power test:			
O_2 intake (l/min)	1.9	3.6	
Ventilation (l/min)	94	98	
Tidal volume (ml)	1500	2900	
Cardiac frequency (beats/min)	192	196	
2. Steady-state test at 60% maximum:			
O_2 intake (ml/min)	1240	2130	
CO_2 output (ml/min)	1300	2120	
Ventilation (l/min)	74	59	
Tidal volume (ml)	1320	2270	
Cardiac frequency (beats/min)	180	174	
Mixed expired PCO_2 (mm Hg)	15	31	
Mixed venous PCO_2 (mm Hg)	61	67	
Arterial PCO_2 (mm Hg)	26	36	
Arterial PO_2 (mm Hg)	61	84	
Arterial pH	7.37	7.35	
VD/VT ratio (%)	0.36	0.11	
A-a PO_2 difference (mm Hg)	62	26	
Venous admixture (%)	10	3	
Cardiac output (l/min)	8.4	17.7	
Plasma lactate (mM/l)	8	3	

Figure 16. O_2 consumption, cardiac output, and pulmonary disease. O_2 pulse—O_2 consumption/pulse rate. O_2 pulse, March = 1.9/192 = 10 mL. O_2 pulse, December = 3.6/196 = 18 mL. Note increase in cardiac output from March to December of 8.4 L to 17.7 L. (Reproduced with permission from Thieme Stratton, Inc. Jones N. In: Hypoxia—Man at Altitude. Georg Thieme Verlag (ed). Sutton, Jones, Houston Thieme-Stratton, Inc., 1982.)

summary, the mechanical properties of the lungs and thorax can profoundly affect cardiac performance. Preload and afterload are most accurately considered in terms of transmural pressures, i.e., intracavitary pressure minus intrapleural pressure (PPL), and PPL is a function of volume and elastic recoil of the lungs and thorax.

References

1. Weibel ER. Morphometry of the Human Lung. Berlin, Springler, 1963.
2. Pedley TJ, Schrofer RC, Sudlow MF. Energy losses and pressure drop in models of human airways. Resp Physiol 1970;9:371.
3. Mead J. Mechanical properties of lungs. Physiol Rev 1961;41:281.
4. Yanof HM, Davis FA. Biomed Electronics. Philadelphia, 1965.
5. Otis AB. Work of breathing. Physiol Rev 1954;34:449–458.
6. Neergard K von. Neue Auffassugen über einen Grundbegriff der Atemmechanik Die Retraktions Kraft der Lunge abhaengig von der Oberflachens pannung in der Alveolen. Z ges exp Med 1929;66:373.
7. Pattle RE. The surface layer of the lung alveoli. Physiol Rev 1965;45:1–17.
8. Clements JA. Pulmonary edema and permeability of alveolar membranes. Arch Environml Health 1961;2:280–283.
9. Brown ES. Isolation and assay of dipalmityl-lecithin in lung extracts. Am J Physiol 1964;207:402–406.
10. Goerke J, Clements JA. Alveolar surface tension and lung surfactant. In: Handbook of Physiol, Section The Respiratory System, Vol III, Part 1. American Physiological Society, 1986, pp. 247–261.
11. Permutt S, Bromberger-Barnea B, Bane HN. Alveolar pressure pulmonary venous pressure and the vascular waterfall. Med Thoracalis 1962;19:239–260.
12. Permutt S, Riley RL. Hemodynamics of collapsible vessels with tone. The vascular waterfall. J Appl Physiol 1963;18:924–932.
13. Hughes JMB, Glazier JB, Maloney JE, et al. Effect of lung volume or distribution of pulmonary blood flow in man. Respir Physiol 1968;4:58–72.
14. Graham R, Skoog C, Macedo W, et al. Dopamine dobutamine, and phentolamine effects on pulmonary vascular mechanics. J Appl Physiol 1983;54:1277–1283.
15. Thomash J, Griffe ZJ, Roos A. Effects of negative pressure inflation of the lung on pulmonary vascular resistance. J Appl Physiol 1961;16:451–456.
16. Burton AC, Patel DJ. Effects of negative pressure inflation of the lung on pulmonary vascular resistance. J Appl Physiol 1958;12:239.
17. Whittenberger JL, McGregor M, Berglund E, et al. Influence of state of inflation of the lung on pulmonary vascular resistance. J Appl Physiol 1960;15:878–882.
18. Grant BJB. Functional aspects of pulmonary vascular anatomy. In: Dantzker. Cardiopulmonary Critical Care, Second Edition. Saunders, 1991.
19. Vischer MB, Rupp A, Scott FH. Lung inflation and pulmonary vascular resistance. Am J Physiol 1924;70:585.

20. Hyatt RE, Wilcox RE. The pressure flow relationship of the intrathoracic airway in man. J Clin Invest 1963;42:29–39.
21. Guyton AC, Lindsey AW, Abernathy JR, et al. Venous return at various right atrial pressures and the normal venous return curve. Am J Physiol 1957;189: 609–614.
22. Guyton AC, Jones CE, Coleman TG. Circulatory Physiology: Cardiac Output and Its Regulation. Philadelphia, WB Saunders, 1973.
23. Starling EH. Linacre Lecture on the Law of the Heart, Cambridge, 1915. New York, Longmans, Green & Co., 1918.
24. Katz AM. The descending limb of the starling curve and the failing heart. Circulation 1965;32:871–875.
25. Sarnoff SJ. Myocardial contractility as described by ventricular function curves: Observations on Starling's law of the heart. Physiol Rev 1955;35:107–122.
26. Kollef MH, Pluss J. Mancardiogenic pulmonary edema following upper airways obstruction. Medicine 1991;70:91–98.
27. Permutt S. Relation between pulmonary arterial pressure and pleural pressure during the acute asthmatic attack. Chest 1973;63(Suppl):25S–28S.
28. Khaja F, Parker JO. Right and left performance in COLD. Am Heart J 1971; 82:319–327.
29. Sagawa K, Suga H, Shoukas AA, et al. Endsystolic pressure-volume ratio. A new index of contractility. Am J Cardiol 1977;40:748–753.
30. Marsh JD, Green LH, Cohn PF, et al. Left ventricular end systolic pressure dimension and stress length relation in normal human subjects. Am J Cardiol 1979;44:1311.
31. Mehmel HC, Stockins B, Ruffman K, et al. The lineacity of the end systolic pressure volume relation in man and its sensitivity for the assessment of LV function. Circulation 1981;63:1216.
32. Sasayama S, Lotoura H. Echocardiographic approach for the clinical assessment of LV function. Jpn Circulation J 1979;43:357.
33. MacNee W. Right ventricular function in cor pulmonale. Cardiology 1988; 75(Suppl 1):30–40.
34. Jardin F, Farcot JC, Boisante L, et al. Influence of positive end expiratory pressure on LV performance. New Engl J Med 1981;304:387–392.
35. Geef RT. Interpretation of pulmonary artery wedge pressure when PEEP is used. Anesthesiology 1977;46:383–384.
36. Downs JA, Douglas ME. Assessment of cardiac filling pressures during continuous positive pressure ventilation. Crit Care Med 1980;8:285–290.
37. Smiseth OA, Refsam H, Tyberg JV. Pericardial pressure assessed by right atrial pressure: A basis for calculation of LV transmural pressure. Am Heart J 1984;108:603–605.
38. Pinsky M, Vincent JL, deSweet JM. Estimating left ventricular filling pressure during positive end expiratory pressure in humans. Am Rev Resp Dis 1991;143: 25–31.
39. Butler J, Albert RK. Estimating LV filling pressure in patients receiving PEEP. Am Rev Resp Dis 1991;143:993–994.
40. Marini JJ, O'Quin R, Culver BH, et al. Estimation of transmural cardiac pressures during ventilation with PEEP. J Appl Physiol 1982;53(2):384–391.
41. Cournand A, Motley HL, Werk L, et al. Physiological studies of the effects of intermittent positive pressure breathing on cardiac output in man. Am J Physiol 1948;152:162–174.

42. Mathru M, et al. Hemodynamic responses to changes in ventilatory patterns in patients with normal and poor LV reserve. Crit Care Med 1982;10:423–426.
43. Robotham JL, Lixfield W, Holland L, et al. The effects of PEEP on right and left ventricular performance. Am Rev Resp Dis 1980;121:677–683.
44. Viquerat CE, Righetti A, Suter PM. Biventricular volumes and function in patients with adult respiratory distress syndrome ventilated with PEEP. Chest 1983;83(3):509–514.
45. Terai C, Uenishi M, Sugimoto H, et al. Transesophageal echocardiographic dimensional analysis of four cardiac chambers during positive end-expiratory pressure. Anesthesiology 1985;63:640–646.
46. Potkin RT, Hudson LD, Weaver LJ, et al. Effect of positive end-expiratory pressure on right and left ventricular function in patients with the adult respiratory distress syndrome. Am Rev Respir Dis 1987;135:307–311.
47. Fessler H, Brouer RG, Wise RA, et al. Effects of PEEP on the gradient for venous return. Am Rev Resp Dis 1991;143:19–24.
48. Scharf SM, Ingram RH Jr. Influence of abdominal pressure and sympathetic vasoconstriction on the cardiovascular response to PEEP. Am Rev Resp Dis 1977;116:661–670.
49. Braunwald E, Binion JT, Morgan WL Jr, et al. Alterations in central blood volume and cardiac output induced by positive pressure breathing and counteracted by metaraminol. Circ Res 1957;5:670–675.
50. Fessler HE, Brouer RG, Shapiro EP, et al. Effects of PEEP and body position on the thoracic great veins. Am Rev Resp Dis 1993;148:1657–1664.
51. Fessler H, Permutt S. Interaction between the circulatory and ventilatory pumps. In: Roussos C (ed). The Thorax. M Decker, 1995.
52. Emerson H. Artificial respiration in the treatment of edema of the lungs; A suggestion based on animal experimentation. Arch Int Med 1909;3:368–371.
53. Barach AL, Martin J, Eckman M. Positive pressure respiration and its application to the treatment of acute pulmonary edema. Ann Int Med 1938;12:754–795.
54. Rizk NW, Murray JF. PEEP and pulmonary edema. Am J Med 1982;72:381–383.
55. Grace MP, Greenbaum DM. Cardiac performance in response to PEEP in patient with cardiac dysfunction. Crit Care Med 1982;10:358–360.
56. Kussmaul A. Ueber schwielige Mediastino-Pericarditis und den paradoxen. Puls Berl Klin Wochenschr 1983;10:433.
57. Heart Disease. A Textbook of Cardiovascular Medicine. In: Braunwald E. (ed). WB Saunders Co., 1980.
58. McGregor M. Pulsus paradoxus. N Eng J Med 1979;301:480–482.
59. Robotham JL, Lixfeld W, Holland L, et al. Effects of respiration on cardiac performance. J Appl Physiol 1978;44(5):703–709.
60. Robotham JL, Rabson J, Permutt S, et al. Left ventricular hemodynamics during respiration. J Appl Physiol 1979;47(6):1295–1303.
61. Scharf SM, Brown R, Saunders N, et al. Effects of normal and loaded spontaneous inspiration on cardiovascular function. J Appl Physiol 1979;47(3):582–590.
62. Scharf SM. Cardiovascular effects of airways obstruction. Lung 1991;169:1–23.
63. Guz A, Innes JA, Murphy K. Respiratory modulation of left ventricular stroke volume in man measured using pulsed doppler ultrasound. J Physiol 1987;393:499–512.
64. Floyer J. A Treatise of the Asthma, Second Edition London, R Wilkins, 1717.

65. Permutt S. Relation between pulmonary arterial pressure and pleural pressure during the acute asthmatic attack. Chest 1973;63(Suppl):258–285.
66. Jardin F, Farcot JC, Boisante L, et al. Mechanism of pyridoxic pulse in bronchial asthma. Circulation 1982;66(4):887–894.
67. Shabetai R, Mangiardi L, Bhargava V, et al. The pericardium and cardiac function. Prog Cardiovasc Dis 1979;22:107.
68. Montes de Oca M, Rassulo J, Celli B. Relationship between O_2 pulse and intrathoracic pressure in COPD patients. Chest 1995;108:155S.
69. Nery LE, Wasserman K, French W, et al. Contrasting cardiovascular and respiratory responses to exercise in mitral valve and chronic obstructive pulmonary diseases. Chest 1983;83:446–453.
70. Butler J, Schrijen A, Henriquez JM, et al. Cause of the raised wedge pressure on exercise in COPD. An Rev Resp Dis 1988;138:350–354.
71. Jones N. In: Georg Thieme Verlag (ed). Hypoxia—Man at Altitude. Sutton, Jones, Houston Thieme-Stratton, Inc., 1982.

Chapter 2

Mechanisms for the Formation and Reabsorption of Pulmonary Edema

Michael A. Matthay, M.D., Frederick A. Tibayan

The overall objective of this chapter is to consider the mechanisms that are responsible for the formation and the resolution of pulmonary edema. Several experimental and clinical studies have examined the pathophysiologic basis for the formation of pulmonary edema. In general, the etiology of pulmonary edema is divided into high pressure (hydrostatic) or increased permeability. However, there is evidence that in some circumstances these distinctions do not adequately describe the pathogenesis of pulmonary edema. There is evidence that both hydrostatic and increased permeability may contribute to the development of pulmonary edema in some clinical conditions. Therefore, the first part of this chapter will discuss the formation of pulmonary edema with a review of the classic distinction between hydrostatic and increased permeability, but will also consider conditions where both mechanisms may contribute to the development of pulmonary edema. The second section of the chapter will consider the development of pulmonary edema from both increased hydrostatic pressure and increased lung vascular permeability. The third part of the chapter will review new evidence regarding the resolution of pulmonary edema. In the last 10 years, there has been an impressive increase in our basic understanding of the mechanisms of the resolution of alveolar edema. These new developments will be reviewed.

From: Cosentino AM, Martin RJ (eds.): Cardiothoracic Interrelationships in Clinical Practice. © Futura Publishing Co., Inc., Armonk, NY, 1997.

Formation of Pulmonary Edema

In order to understand the formation of pulmonary edema, the structural and physiologic basis for the exchange of fluid and protein in the lung must be considered. First, this section will deal with the morphology of the blood-gas barrier, including the microvascular barrier, the interstitial space, and the alveolar barrier. Second, the Starling equation, which describes the movement of liquid and protein across these semi-permeable barriers, will be considered. This equation also provides a means of classifying pulmonary edema into two types: edema resulting from increased microvascular pressure; and edema resulting from increased permeability. Finally, the pathophysiology of high pressure edema, both interstitial and alveolar, along with a discussion of the possible role of increased permeability from high vascular pressures, will close this section.

The Structural Basis of Pulmonary Edema

Most of the available evidence indicates that the major function of protein and fluid exchange occurs in the microvessels of the lung. On the arterial side, these vessels are without media and adventitia, consisting of only endothelial and basal lamina, measuring <75 µm in diameter. On the venous side, the microvessels can be up to 200 µm in diameter, also made up of endothelium and basal lamina. The thicker walls and relatively lower total surface area probably prevent any meaningful exchange across the larger vessels.

The capillaries in the lung are surrounded by the alveolar space and the interstitial space (Figure 1). Normally, the barrier has a thin side, where the capillary endothelium and the alveolar epithelium are attenuated and their basement membranes are fused. This reduces the distance of gas diffusion to 1 µm or less. The opposite side of the barrier is the "thick" side. Here, the endothelium and epithelium are not attenuated, and the basement membranes are not fused. Ground substance, cells, and connective tissue fibrils are found on this side.[1]

Figure 1. Electron photomicrograph of a human lung. Two capillaries containing red blood cells (RBC) are suspended in the interalveolar septum between two alveolar spaces (AS). The basement membranes (BM) of the epithelium (EP) and endothelium (EN) appear to be fused over the thin portion of the septum (or air-blood barrier) and are separated over the thick portion of the septum containing the interstitial space (IS). Note the endothelial junction (J), which is normal in this micrograph (in contrast to Figure 2). Horizontal bar = 1 um. Magnification × 11,000. (Reprinted with permission from Murray JF (ed). The Normal Lung. Philadelphia, PA, W.B. Saunders Company, 1976, p. 136.)

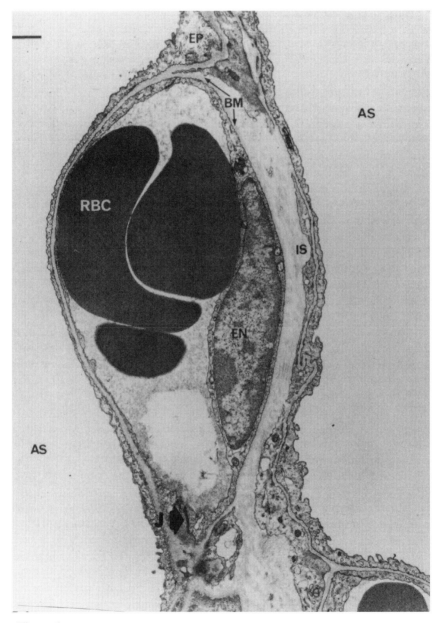

Figure 1.

Interstitial edema collects primarily on the thick side of the barrier, and this is where most endothelial cell junctions are found. Physiologic movement of proteins and fluid probably occurs through these intercellular junctions.[2] To support this theory, freeze-fracture studies have shown that endothelial cell junctions are relatively leaky.[3] In fact, some of these junctions can be opened by very high distending pressures.[2] Of course, other pathways exist for the passage of fluid, and protein, but they are not likely to contribute significantly.

After filtration through the microvascular barrier, the fluid and proteins enter the interstitial space of the lung. The interstitium of the alveolar walls differs from that of the extra-alveolar space in at least two ways that influence the movement of filtered fluid. First, lymphatic vessels are not found in the alveolar walls, but occur only in the loose connective tissue of the peribronchovascular cuffs, interlobular septa, and pleura. Second, although the compartments are continuous, the hydrostatic pressure of the extra-alveolar interstitial space is negative relative to the pressure in the alveolar wall interstitium. This was proposed separately by Howell et al.[4] and Staub et al.,[5] and later confirmed by Battacharya and Staub[6] with micropuncture of the interstitium around alveolar walls, arterioles, venules, and the hilum. This pressure gradient allows the loose connective tissue spaces to serve as sumps for the alveolar wall interstitium, draining fluid proximally towards the peribronchovascular spaces.

The loose connective tissue spaces are also very distensible. This allows them to collect a large volume of fluid without a large rise in interstitial pressure. Even while containing a substantial volume of fluid, a pressure gradient still exists in the interstitium, and edema fluid can drain toward the hilum from the alveolar interstitial space. This prevents a rise in pressure in the alveolar walls, which could result in alveolar edema. Gee and William[7] have shown that the bronchovascular cuffs are able to hold up to 500 mL in this capacity. The fluid in the extra-alveolar spaces is in turn drained by the lymphatics running through them. Normally, the lymph vessels return all filtered fluid to systemic circulation at the rate of 10–20 mL/hour.[5]

Under normal conditions, and even in the early phase of pulmonary edema, fluid in the alveolar wall interstitium does not cross the epithelium into the alveolar space unless the barrier has been damaged. The alveolar barrier consists of two primary cell types. Flat, attenuated type I cells are less numerous but cover 95% of the total surface area of the alveolar space. Rounded, surfactant-producing type II cells are greater in number, but cover much less area. These cells are arranged in a single cell layer. Although the alveolar barrier is very thin, the junctions between the cells are extremely tight. These non-leaky tight junctions give the alveolar epithelium very low permeability to fluid, proteins, and even small solutes.[8] Thus, there can be considerable fluid accumulation in the interstitium without the development of alveolar edema.

The Physiologic Basis of Pulmonary Edema

Movement of fluid and proteins through the pulmonary endothelium is believed to obey the Starling equation. The Starling equation predicts that the net filtration of fluid and proteins across a semi-permeable barrier is the product of the driving pressure and the conductance, or permeability, of the barrier. The total driving pressure is the sum of the hydrostatic and osmotic pressures. Thus:

$$QF = K[(Pmv - Ppmv) - \sigma(\Pi mv - \Pi pmv)]$$

In this equation, Qf is the net filtration rate, K is the filtration coefficient or the conductance across the barrier, Pmv stands for the microvascular hydrostatic pressure, Ppmv for the hydrostatic pressure of the perimicrovascular space, Πmv is the microvascular osmotic pressure, and Πpmv is the osmotic pressure of the perimicrovascular space. The reflection coefficient, σ, indicates the effectiveness of the osmotic pressure difference across the barrier. For example, if σ were equal to one, the barrier would be totally impermeable to protein molecules. On the other hand, a reflection coefficient of zero would indicate that the barrier is freely permeable to proteins. In the lung, σ is estimated to be around 0.9 for the endothelial barrier and very close to 1 for the alveolar epithelium.[2] These values are consistent with the structural studies previously mentioned, in which the endothelial cell junctions were found to be relatively leaky, while those of the alveolar epithelium are very tight.

The Starling equation fails to account for two factors affecting fluid and protein exchange in the lung. First, fluid balance depends on the function of the lymphatics, which remove much of the fluid that is filtered across the microvascular barrier. If the lymphatics are blocked, pulmonary edema results. Second, fluid and protein exchange depend on the surface of filtration and the perfused vascular surface area in the lung can change under pathologic or normal conditions, as in the recruitment of vessels during exercise. An increase in surface area can lead to increase in lung lymph flow without changing any of the variables in the Starling equation.[9]

In clinical practice, pulmonary edema is classified into two types by using the Starling equation: high-pressure or increased-permeability pulmonary edema. These headings are not mutually exclusive, and cases of increased permeability can be complicated by an increase in hydrostatic pressure. Also, it is possible that some extreme cases of hydrostatic pressure edema may be complicated by increased permeability edema. For purposes of initial explanation, however, the two types will be considered separately, and then the clinical conditions in which a combination of hydrostatic and increased permeability mechanisms will be considered.

High Pressure Pulmonary Edema

The Starling equation predicts that high-pressure pulmonary edema will develop from a large increase in the difference between microvascular and perimicrovascular hydrostatic pressures. This often arises in the context of left-sided congestive heart failure,[10] but can also result from pulmonary venous hypertension.[11] Theoretically, a drop in lung interstitial pressure should also lead to high-pressure edema; and this concept has received some support by studies in dogs' lungs.[12,13]

As hydrostatic pressure increases in the microvasculature of the lung, the rate of filtration increases. Note, however, that the reflection coefficient of the endothelium is quite high (about 0.9), and that even in severe edema, the protein content of the edema fluid is less than that of plasma. The filtrate in the alveolar wall flows down a pressure gradient into the loose connective tissue of the bronchovascular cuffs. This extra-alveolar interstitium is very distensible, and can collect a large volume of fluid without a significant increase in pressure.[2] Figure 2 is the picture of interstitial edema, which can cause dyspnea and is detectable on radiograph, but does not interfere with gas exchange because no alveolar flooding occurs.[14]

Several safety factors attenuate the development and progression of pulmonary edema. As already mentioned, a functional lymphatic system is a crucial safeguard. The lymphatics drain off fluid from the interstitial space and prevent a rise in perimicrovascular hydrostatic pressure that might lead to alveolar flooding (Figure 3). Second, even if the lymph vessels cannot keep up with fluid formation, the loose connective tissue of the peribronchovascular cuffs can hold 500 mL of edema fluid.[5,10] Third, when fluid filters through the microvascular barrier, it dilutes the protein in the interstitium, reducing the osmotic pressure. Following the Starling equation, this would lead to a greater tendency for fluid to flow into the vessels, since plasma has a relatively high protein content. The lowering of the perimicrovascular osmotic pressure probably offsets about half of the increase in microvascular hydrostatic pressure.[15] Finally, although the peribronchovascular cuffs are very distensible, some finite increase in interstitial hydrostatic pressure must occur that would at least partly diminish the pressure gradient from the vessels to the interstitium.

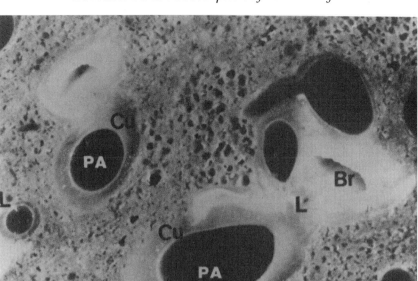

Figure 2. Photograph of a frozen sheep lung. In this experimental study, left atrial pressure was elevated to 22 m H_2O for 4 hours. The result is interstitial pulmonary edema with perivascular fluid cuffs (Cu) around pulmonary arteries (PA) and small airways (Br) that are approximately 2–3 mm in diameter. There are also some lymphatics (L) visible in the fluid cuffs also. (Reproduced with permission from George RB(ed). Chest Medicine. New York, Churchill Livingstone, 1983.)

When the edema fluid exceeds the capacity of the interstitial space, a change in the alveolar barrier occurs and fluid enters the air spaces, resulting in alveolar edema.[10] The sites of flooding into the air spaces, as well as the precise changes in the epithelial tight junctions, are as yet unknown. Channels in the terminal airway epithelium as well as the alveolar barrier may play a part. However, when alveolar flooding occurs, the reflection coefficient of the epithelium changes from one to zero, and the barrier is freely permeable to liquid and protein. Experimental studies have demonstrated that edema fluid in the interstitium and the alveolar spaces have the same protein content.[16,17]

Most of the pathophysiologic changes that have been observed with high-pressure pulmonary edema follow logically from the flooding of the air spaces. The fluid in the alveoli prevents ventilation and causes ventilation-perfusion mismatch or shunt, depending on the extent of flooding. The edema fluid in the alveoli may inactivate some of the surfactant and can result in atelectasis, increasing the amount of shunt. Experimental studies of high-pressure edema have shown that alveolar flooding corresponds

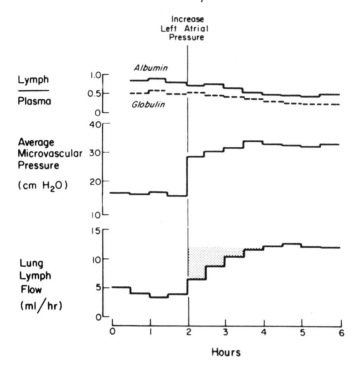

Figure 3. Time course of the effect of increased pulmonary microvascular pressure on lung lymph flow and the lymph-to-plasma protein concentration ratios in unanesthetized sheep. After 2 hours of baseline study, left atrial pressure was elevated by inflating a chronically implanted balloon. Note the rise in lymph flow is more than double baseline values, and the lymph-to-plasma concentration falls. (Reproduced with permission from the American Heart Association in Circ Res 1975;37:273.)

with a decrease in arterial oxygenation and an increase in the alveolar-arterial oxygen difference.[14]

Increased Permeability Pulmonary Edema

The Starling equation predicts that a change in the permeability of the microvascular membrane will result in a marked increase in the amount of fluid and protein that leaves the vascular space and enters the interstitium of the lung. Pulmonary edema fluid of this type should have a high protein concentration because the vascular membrane no longer has the capacity to restrict the outward movement of large molecules such as plasma proteins. The results of a number of studies have confirmed that the alveolar edema fluid has a high protein concentration (80% or higher) compared with the plasma protein concentration.[18–20]

Experimentally, a variety of agents have been used to injure the lung, some given by the intravenous route and others directly into the air spaces of the lung. Severe hemorrhagic edema is produced in sheep or dogs when oleic acid is injected in doses of 0.08 mL/kg body weight.[21] Intravenous alloxan has been used in dogs as a means of producing a severe pulmonary edema. In order to stimulate the effects of gastric aspiration, instillation of hydrochloric acid via the airways has been used experimentally to produce combined epithelial and endothelial injury.[22] One of the limitations of all these experimental approaches to injuring the lung is that they are severe and produce changes that are not reversible and are therefore suitable for acute studies only. Some investigators have been able to reduce the severity of injury by lowering the dose (particularly of oleic acid) to sublethal doses that allow unanesthetized animals to be studied for a few days.

One useful experimental approach for producing reversible acute lung injury has been achieved with intravenous air emboli[23] or *E. coli* endotoxin in unanesthetized spontaneously breathing sheep.[24] Both these means of producing acute lung injury have allowed investigators to study the early phase of acute lung injury.

In the *E. coli* endotoxin model of acute lung injury, there is an early rise in pulmonary artery pressure with an abrupt rise in lymph flow accompanied by a decrease in the lymph-to-plasma protein concentration ratio (Figure 4). This pattern is similar to the effect of left atrial hypertension on lymph flow (Figure 3), suggesting that the elevated pulmonary artery pressure is transmitted to fluid exchanging vessels in the lung. After 1–2 hours of *E. coli* endotoxin infusion, the pulmonary artery pressure declines (but not to baseline levels) and the lung lymph flow rises to very high levels in association with a rise in the lymph protein concentration and a return of the lymph-to-plasma protein concentration ratio to baseline levels. This is the classic pattern of increased permeability pulmonary edema.

Venous air emboli given to sheep produces a rise in pulmonary vascular pressures, a marked increase in lymph flow, and no change in the lymph-to-plasma protein concentration ratios.[23] Since the air emboli actually decrease lung surface area for filtration, the unchanged lymph-to-plasma protein concentration ratio indicating a significant increase in lung vascular permeability. In both endotoxin- and air emboli-induced lung injury, interstitial edema and mild hypoxemia develop in parallel with the increase in lymph flow. Both forms of acute lung injury are partially mediated by neutrophils, perhaps in part by the release of toxic oxygen radicals from degranulated neutrophils. These physiologic studies have been complemented

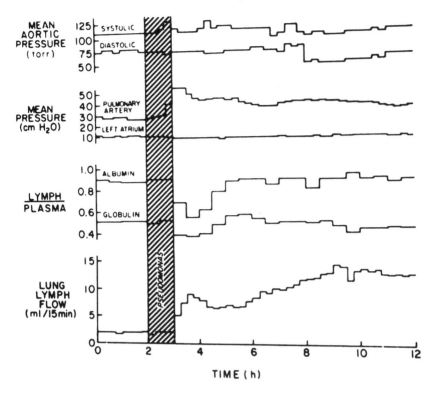

Figure 4. Effects of infusion of *Pseudomonas aeruginosa* on lung vascular pressures, lymph flow, and lymph-to-plasma protein concentration in unanesthetized sheep. Note that there is an initial rise in lymph flow associated with a fall in the lymph-to-plasma protein concentration ratio when pulmonary artery pressure had doubled. Then, there is a later, more dramatic increase in lung lymph flow with a return of the lymph-to-plasma protein concentration ratios to baseline levels when the pulmonary artery pressure has returned toward baseline levels. This is the late phase of increased vascular permeability with protein-rich lymph. A similar response occurs with *E. coli* endotoxin. (Reproduced with permission from The Journal of Clinical Investigation, 1974;92:1225.)

by morphologic studies to determine the ultrastructural basis for the increased-permeability pulmonary edema. Interestingly, the primary vascular lesions are located in different portions of the pulmonary circulation.

In some experimental studies, it has been difficult to determine whether an increase in the lung lymph flow develops because of a change in vascular permeability or an increase in the perfused vascular surface area. One approach to differentiating an increase in vascular permeability from an increase in surface area is to increase microvascular pressure and follow the lymph-to-plasma protein concentration ratios. For example, Ohkuda et al.,[23] demonstrated that after venous air emboli were given to sheep, left atrial pressure elevations resulted in a further rise in lymph flow but no decline in the lymph-to-plasma protein concentration ratio, demonstrating that the primary lesion was an increase in vascular permeability.

In contrast, when left atrial pressure elevation results in a decline in the lymph-to-plasma protein concentration ratio (Figure 3), it is likely that a major change in vascular permeability has not occurred. For example, a study from our laboratory was designed to test the overperfusion theory of pulmonary edema and determine if high blood flow to a restricted portion of the lung with and without hypoxia would result in a high pressure or an increased-vascular permeability pulmonary edema.[25] Anesthetized sheep were prepared surgically so that pulmonary and systemic hemodynamics and lung lymph flow could be measured, then 65% of the lung mass was resected. There was a substantial rise in lymph flow from the remaining lung with a small decrease in the lymph-to-plasma protein concentration ratio. In order to be certain that there was no significant change in permeability, left atrial pressure was elevated with and without hypoxia. The results consistently showed a further rise in lymph flow that was accompanied by a marked decrease in the lymph-to-plasma protein ratio. These results indicated that the endothelial barrier continued to restrict the movement of macromolecules, suggesting that the increase in lymph flow was related to high pressure alone and not to an increase in permeability.

Pulmonary Edema that Develops from Both Increased Hydrostatic Pressure and Increased Vascular Permeability

Several studies, both clinical and experimental, have suggested that in some cases, increased hydrostatic pressure in the microcirculation can injure the endothelium, increasing its permeability. Very high pressures resulting from left ventricular failure and the dynamic effect of blood flowing through a restricted vascular bed at high velocity, resulting from pulmonary emboli or resection and transfusion, have been proposed as mechanisms for physically injuring the endothelial barrier.[26,27] It is thought that this stress on the vascular walls could open the intercellular junctions. However, as described in the prior section, by overperfusing the lungs of sheep, we found that high pressure and increased flow through a restricted vascular bed resulted in hydrostatic pulmonary edema, but not an increase in vascular permeability.[25] However, some recent studies have raised the possibility that elevated hydrostatic vascular pressures may indeed result in injury to the microcirculation.

For example, work from the laboratory of Bachofen and colleagues[28,29] indicated that epithelial lesions can be found in isolated perfused lungs ventilated with positive pressure when vascular pressures were raised to markedly elevated levels. Interestingly, the morphologic studies indicated that there was regional distribution of hydrostatic pulmonary edema that was not entirely accounted for by gravity dependence. Pulmonary edema within one lung was found to be inhomogenous and changes in alveolar architecture occurred with bulging of alveolar capillaries apparently due to loss of air-liquid surface tension. There were significant epithelial lesions that seemed to occur in areas where the pulmonary capillary endothelium was not apparently injured. One criticism of the studies is that the technique for preparation of the lungs for histologic analysis was done by vascular fixation so that pressures were returned to normal before the fixatives were injected. Bachofen and colleagues interpreted their findings as indicating that elevated vascular pressures with elevated interstitial edema caused the epithelial lesions.

There are also some recent studies from the laboratory of West and associates[30] indicating that high perfusion and inflation pressures can cause endothelial lesions. Their studies showed a direct relationship between the number of endothelial cell lesions and the levels of both lung perfusion and lung inflation.[30,31] These studies raise the possibility that hydrostatic stress may cause endothelial injury, although the actual model for the studies is not entirely physiologic. Nevertheless, these studies do raise the intriguing possibility that under some conditions hydrostatic stress may cause lung endothelial and pulmonary epithelial lesions.

Are there any clinical circumstances under which pulmonary edema may form that might be modeled by the mechanisms explored in these studies? Two obvious candidates are high altitude pulmonary edema and neurogenic pulmonary edema.[27] High altitude pulmonary edema is known to be associated with markedly elevated pulmonary vascular pressures and it may be that regional overperfusion occurs in the presence of hypoxia with injury to the capillary endothelium and/or epithelium occurring in some portions of the lung.[32] Firm evidence supporting this hypothesis is still not available, but it is certainly a reasonable possibility. In this circumstance, lowering of vascular pressures should prevent or attenuate the development of pulmonary edema. A recent study that showed that nifedipine could prevent the development of high altitude pulmonary edema in mountain climbers who had previously experienced high altitude pulmonary edema suggests that this may be a reasonable explanation.[33]

Neurogenic pulmonary edema has been studied experimentally and clinically.[34] The results have indicated that in some cases animals develop a hydrostatic pulmonary edema with a low protein concentration in the edema fluid while in other cases, there is an increased permeability edema with a high protein concentration. A recent clinical study from our institution found that patients with neurogenic pulmonary edema had a hydrostatic profile in 60% of the cases and an increased permeability profile in the other 40% of cases.[35] It is possible that the primary hydrostatic lesion may be related to pulmonary venoconstriction, a mechanism that has been explored experimentally. Although for years there was a major interest in the possibility that transient elevations of pulmonary vascular pressures might cause permeability lesions in the human pulmonary circulation in neurogenic edema, human studies have not specifically supported this hypothesis, although more work needs to be done. In any case, it is possible that in some cases neurogenic edema may represent also a combination of both hydrostatic and increased vascular permeability in the lung.

How often is increased permeability pulmonary edema complicated by elevations in hydrostatic pressure? It has been recognized for many years that an increase in lung vascular permeability can be complicated by elevations in pulmonary microvascular pressure. Several animal studies demonstrated that elevations of hydrostatic pressure above normal will markedly increase the quantity of edema fluid that enters the extravascular space of the lung in the presence of an increase in lung vascular permeability.[36–38] Clinical studies have suggested that this certainly occurs in some patients.[38] Thus, while the primary lesion might be related to an increase in lung vascular permeability, the mechanism of pulmonary edema clinically may be related to both elevations of hydrostatic pressure and an increase in lung vascular permeability.

Work from our own laboratory suggests that there are patients who have a pulmonary edema fluid to plasma protein concentration that is midway between criteria for hydrostatic edema and criteria for increased permeability. In general, hydrostatic edema is defined as a edema fluid total protein to plasma ratio <0.65 and increased permeability is defined as ratio >0.75. We have found that somewhere between 10%–15% of patients will have an initial edema fluid to plasma protein concentration ratio between 0.65–0.75, suggesting that they may have a combination of a mild increase in vascular permeability possibly complicated by a modest elevation in pulmonary vascular pressures.[19] In some cases of hydrostatic pulmonary edema, there are significant numbers of alveolar neurophils, a finding that may relate to proinflammatory factors in the air spaces of the lung.[39]

Is it necessary to abandon the traditional classification of pulmonary edema as either hydrostatic or increased permeability? I believe the answer is no. Most cases of pulmonary edema can be correctly classified clinically as either hydrostatic or increased permeability. However, there may well be

10%–15% of cases in which both mechanisms are present and contribute to the development of pulmonary edema. Further clinical and experimental studies may help to identify this particular overlap group.

Resolution of Pulmonary Edema

Once the air spaces have flooded with edema fluid from the interstitium of the lung, what are the mechanisms available for removal of the excess fluid? In order to address this issue, several years ago we instilled a protein solution (autologous serum or plasma or 5% albumin in Ringer's lactate) into the distal air spaces of sheep, and then measured the removal of this fluid from the air spaces. Since protein is removed from the air spaces of the lung very slowly because of the normally tight alveolar epithelial barrier,[40] we were able to use the concentration of protein in the air spaces as an indicator of alveolar fluid clearance. Interestingly, the concentration of protein in the air spaces progressively increased to levels well above the plasma protein concentration.[41,42] Over time, the alveolar protein concentration increased in proportion to the removal of the liquid volume from the air spaces and the lung as a whole (Table 1). These observations in sheep led us to propose that the process of alveolar fluid clearance required an active ion transport process.[40] In subsequent clinical studies, we found the same pattern of protein concentration of alveolar edema fluid during the resolution of pulmonary edema in patients (Table 2).[43]

_____ **Table 1** _____

Alveolar Liquid Clearance in Sheep as Reflected by Progressive Concentration of Protein in the Air Spaces of the Lung

| Time (hours) | Alveolar Protein Concentration (g/100 mL) | | Lung Liquid Clearance (% of Instilled) |
	Initial[a]	Final[b]	
4	6.3 ± 0.6	8.4 ± 0.6	33.2
12	5.9 ± 0.4	10.2 ± 1.2	59.2
24	6.4 ± 0.6	12.9 ± 1.9	75.9

Data shown as mean ± SD.

[a]The protein concentration of the instilled serum (3 mL/kg).

[b]The increase in concentration of protein in the air spaces can be used to estimate the alveolar liquid clearance by a simple proportion calculation since we know the instilled volume and the initial and final alveolar protein concentration. Data collected from references 40 and 41.

_____ **Table 2**_____

Resolution of Alveolar Edema in Patients with Acute Pulmonary Edema

Classification of Edema	Number	Total Protein Concentration (g/100 mL) Initial	Final
Hydrostatic	15	3.3 ± 1.0	4.8 ± 2.3[a]
↑Permeability	9	4.7 ± 0.9	6.8 ± 1.6[a]

Data as mean ± SD.
[a]P < 0.05 compared to initial sample.
All final alveolar edema fluid samples collected within 12 hours of initial sample?
Data collected from references 43.

Mechanisms of Alveolar Fluid Clearance

Subsequent in vivo studies from our laboratory and studies from other laboratories have confirmed that the process of alveolar fluid reabsorption requires an active process and does not depend on lung inflation or the transpulmonary pressure. For example, in studies in both sheep and dogs, the mode of ventilation (positive pressure or spontaneous) did not alter the rate of alveolar liquid clearance.[36–38] In addition, even the removal of all ventilation did not alter the rate of alveolar fluid clearance.[44] In order to provide direct evidence for the role of sodium transport in the process of alveolar fluid reabsorption in vivo, we found that alveolar fluid reabsorption in sheep[45] and rabbits[46] could be inhibited with amiloride, an inhibitor of apical sodium channel uptake, as well as by ouabain, an inhibitor of Na, K-ATPase enzyme activity.[44] In vitro studies of alveolar epithelial type II cells in monolayers as well as studies in Ussing chambers have demonstrated that these cells actively transport sodium from the apical to the basal surface.[47–49] Thus, the current evidence indicates that the process of alveolar fluid reabsorption depends on sodium uptake into channels on the apical membrane of alveolar type II cells with subsequent active extrusion of the sodium to the basolateral interstitial space by the Na, K-ATPase pump.[50,51] Water crosses the alveolar barrier to maintain isoosmolar conditions, probably by specific proteinaceous water transporters (CHIP 28) that have just recently been identified[52] and described in the alveolar epithelium.[53] Our current understanding of the basic ion and water transport processes responsible for alveolar fluid reabsorption are summarized in Figure 5.

It is important to also emphasize that several experimental studies from our laboratory as well as other investigators have indicated that basal

ALVEOLAR LIQUID REABSORPTION
DEPENDS ON ACTIVE NA$^+$ TRANSPORT

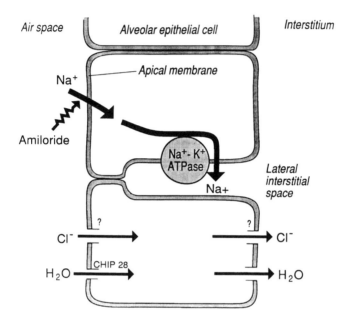

Figure 5. Schematic drawing of our current understanding of the mechanisms for alveolar fluid reabsorption. The alveolar or air space side is designated on the left, the alveolar epithelial cells in the middle, and the lung interstitial space on the right. Sodium (Na$^+$) is taken up by amiloride sensitive channels on the apical surface of alveolar epithelial type II cells and then actively pumped out into the interstitial space by the Na, K-ATPase pumps on the basolateral surface of the cells. Then, chloride (Cl$^-$) probably follows by an incompletely characterized transcellular pathway, which maintains electrical neutrality. Water (H$_2$O) follows probably by a predominant transcellular route through specific water channels, some of which are currently designated CHIP 28. (Reproduced with permission from Williams and Wilkins in New Horizons: The Science and Practice of Acute Medicine 1993;1:616.)

alveolar fluid clearance can be accelerated by beta adrenergic agonist therapy. We have found an impressive increase in alveolar liquid clearance in our in vivo studies in sheep,[54] dogs,[42] and rats,[55] although rabbits do not respond to beta adrenergic agonists.[45] Other investigators have also found an impressive increase in sodium transport in isolated alveolar type II cells[56] as well as in the isolated perfused rat lung.[57] Our most recent work indicates that beta adrenergic agonist therapy increases alveolar liquid clearance in the isolated human lung,[58] suggesting that basal alveolar liquid clearance in humans can be accelerated.

Mechanisms of Alveolar Protein Clearance

What are the mechanisms available for the removal of the excess protein in the air spaces of the lung? Even after flooding of the air spaces in hydrostatic pulmonary edema, a considerable quantity of protein needs to be removed from the air spaces of the lung. Experimental studies from our laboratory have indicated that soluble protein is removed from the air spaces primarily by diffusion between alveolar epithelial cells.[59] The evidence for this conclusion is based in part on clearance of molecules across the epithelium at a rate that is inversely related to molecular size.[60] There is undoubtedly some endocytosis and transcytosis of protein by alveolar epithelial cells, although most of our in vivo studies indicate that this mechanism cannot account for the majority of alveolar protein clearance when large quantities of protein have entered the air spaces of the lung.[59,60] Mucociliary clearance is a minor pathway, as is protein degradation and macrophage engulfment, at least in the uninjured lung.[59] However, in the setting of acute lung injury in which precipitation of protein occurs in the alveoli, the mechanism for removal of excess protein may then include a more important role for alveolar macrophage engulfment and protein degradation.

Mechanisms of Alveolar Epithelial Recovery After Acute Lung Injury

Because of our increased understanding of the role of the alveolar epithelial barrier in regulating fluid and protein balance under normal and abnormal conditions, it was possible to develop methods to monitor the function of the alveolar epithelial barrier. Two well described properties of the alveolar epithelial barrier that can be monitored experimentally are: (1) its relative impermeability to the bidirectional movement of protein; and (2) its capacity to remove excess alveolar fluid from the air spaces of the lung. In several of our experimental studies, alveolar epithelial injury has been quantified by the degree of bidirectional or protein flux across the epithelial barrier; also, the net capacity of the alveolar epithelial barrier to remove excess alveolar fluid has been used as a marker of its overall function.[54,61] Logically, in order to remove excess alveolar fluid, a significant fraction of the alveolar epithelial barrier must be sufficiently intact with normal tight junctions and a functioning sodium transport system.

For example, after severe oleic acid-induced pulmonary edema in sheep, the initial concentration of protein in pulmonary edema was equal to plasma protein concentration, indicating there was a marked increase in protein permeability of both the lung endothelial and alveolar epithelial barriers.[62] In these studies, in spite of the early increase in epithelial permeability following administration of intravenous oleic acid, there was evidence that the epithelial barrier was beginning to recover between 5–8 hours after the oleic acid was given. Alveolar protein concentration had risen to 30% above plasma protein concentration and there was a parallel decline in extravascular lung water, indicating that the epithelial barrier was recovering. Thus, this study demonstrated that the epithelial barrier was capable of recovering soon after severe injury. Similar data is available from studies in which rats were exposed to 100% oxygen for 40 hours, resulting in a 30% increase in extravascular lung water and a modest increase in epithelial protein permeability to protein. However, when fluid was instilled into the air spaces of these rat lungs, the fluid was removed normally and the rats even responded to an exogenous beta adrenergic agonist (terbutaline) with an increase in the rate of alveolar liquid clearance. Thus, in the setting of mild to moderate lung injury or following severe injury, it appears that the alveolar epithelial barrier is capable of removing fluid and providing a barrier to further alveolar flooding. This was also true in a study carried out in sheep over 24 hours in which *P. aeruginosa* pneumonia caused a marked increase in epithelial permeability to protein, but after 24 hours the epithelial barrier had recovered and net alveolar fluid clearance had occurred.[61]

Our clinical studies have been designed to assess the function of the alveolar epithelial barrier in the first 12–24 hours after the onset of acute lung injury. By measuring sequential concentrations of protein in alveolar fluid in patients with acute lung injury, it is possible to determine if fluid is being removed from the air spaces of the lung in spite of the presence of severe acute lung injury and acute respiratory failure. In our initial study, we found that approximately 40% of patients with acute lung injury and increased permeability pulmonary edema were capable of removing some of their excess alveolar fluid within the first 12 hours after injury (Figure 6).[43] This finding indicated that the epithelial barrier was functional and intact, at least to some degree. Interestingly, these patients had a lower mortality and a more rapid recovery from acute respiratory failure than patients who showed no evidence of alveolar fluid clearance in the first 12 hours after acute lung injury. In that particular study, in the patients who showed evidence of alveolar fluid reabsorption, there was no significant difference in their pulmonary arterial wedge pressure, levels of positive end-expiratory pressure and other indices of mechanical ventilation when compared to the patients who had no evidence of alveolar fluid reabsorption. These results suggested that the patients who had no evidence of alveolar fluid protein concentration in the first 12 hours had sufficiently severe endothelial and/or epithelial injury so that net alveolar fluid clearance could not occur. In contrast, the Group A patients who were able to concentrate their

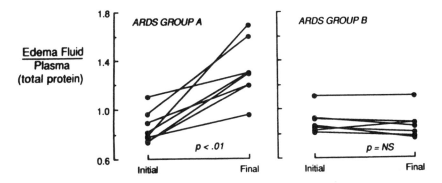

Figure 6. Individual data points are shown for the initial and final pulmonary edema fluid-to-plasma protein concentration ratio in the adult respiratory distress syndrome (ARDS) Group A patients who clinically improved compared to the ARDS Group B patients who did not clinically improve. The time interval between the initial and the final sample was similar between the Group A (6.8±5.1 hours) compared to the Group B (5.4±4.1 hours) patients. Mortality was lower in the Group A patients, suggesting that the early ability to remove some of the alveolar edema fluid indicated an intact alveolar epithelial barrier function with an improved prognosis for recovery. (Reproduced with permission from American Review of Respiratory Disease 1990;142:1254.)

alveolar protein did have evidence of net alveolar fluid reabsorption and a functionally intact and recovering alveolar barrier. In that same study there was evidence of some improvement radiographically in the Group A patients who had a rise in alveolar fluid protein concentration. Thus, this index of alveolar barrier function may be clinically useful as a prognostic index.[43] It is inexpensive, noninvasive, and it is independent of changes in the tidal volume or PEEP, interventions that may improve oxygenation, but not necessarily change the distribution of alveolar edema fluid or the total quantity of pulmonary edema in the lung. Also, it may be useful in several types of acute lung injury, as we recently reported in a case of salt water near-drowning.[63]

The critical role of the alveolar epithelial type II cell in regenerating an intact alveolar wall following acute lung injury has been established in both experimental and clinical studies in vivo.[64] Although alveolar type II cells cover <5% of the total lung surface area, they are responsible for forming a new epithelial barrier following alveolar epithelial type I cell necrosis.[65,66] The factors that promote alveolar wall regeneraton are largely unknown. However, recent studies regarding the mechanisms of wound healing in non-pulmonary epithelial and endothelial cells have demonstrated the importance of extracellular matrix molecules, interaction of cell adhesion molecules, and the autocrine and paracrine action of growth factors in the lung.[66,67]

In order to understand the basic function of the alveolar epithelial type II cell in wound healing, we recently developed an experimental in vitro model in which wound healing can be studied quantitatively.[68] The results indicate that the process of wound healing can be accelerated with TGF-a, a growth factor that is present in the alveolar fluid of patients with acute lung injury.[68] The results also indicate that soluble and insoluble fibronectin accelerates wound healing.

In summary, it is likely that interaction of growth factors cytokines, and extracellular matrix are important in determining the ability of the alveolar epithelial barrier to recover from acute lung injury.[69–71] Much more work is needed to determine the basic mechanisms of repair, as well as to identify why in some patients the process of repair is complicated by a destructive fibrosing alveolitis that results in obliteration of functional air spaces and a loss of vascular supply to the lung.[72]

Acknowledgment: The author wishes to thank Jill Richardson for her assistance in preparing this chapter.

References

1. Staub NC, Albertine KH. Anatomy of the lungs. In: Murray JF, Nadel JA (eds). Textbook of Respiratory Medicine, Second Edition, Volume 1. Philadelphia, PA, WB Saunders Co., 1994, pp. 3–35.
2. Staub NC. The pathogenesis of pulmonary edema. Prog Cardiovasc Dis 1980;23: 53–80.
3. Schneeberger EE, Karnovsky MJ. Substructure of intercellular functions in freeze-fracture alveolar-capillary membranes of mouse lung. Circ Res 1976;38: 404–411.
4. Howell JBL, Permutt S, Proctor DF, et al. Effect of inflation of the lungs on different parts of the pulmonary vascular bed. J Appl Physiol 1961;16:71–76.
5. Staub NC, Nagano H, Pearce MC. Pulmonary edema in dogs, especially the sequence of fluid accumulation in lungs. J Appl Physiol 1967;22:227–240.
6. Battacharya J, Staub NC. Direct measurement of microvascular pressures in the isolated perfused dog lung. Science 1980;210:327–328.
7. Gee MH, William DO. Effect of lung inflation on perivascular cuff fluid volume in isolated dog lung lobes. Microvasc Res 1979;19:209–216.
8. Hastings RH, Grady L, Sakuma T, et al. Clearance of different-sized proteins from the alveolar space in humans. J Appl Physiol 1992;73:1310–1316.
9. Coats G, O'Brodovich H, Jeffries AL, et al. Effects of exercise on lung lymph flow in sheep and goats during normoxia and hypoxia. J Clin Invest 1984;74: 133–141.
10. Matthay MA. Pathophysiology of pulmonary edema. Clin Chest Med 1985;6: 301–314.
11. Hakim TS, Venderzee H, Malik AB. Effects of sympathetic nerve stimulation on lung fluid and protein exchange. J Appl Physiol 1979;47:1025–1030.

12. Albert RK, Lakshminarayan S, Hilkebrandt J, et al. Increased surface tension favors pulmonary edema formation in anesthetized dogs' lungs. J Clin Invest 1979;63:1015–1016.
13. Nieman GF, Bredenberg CE. High surface tension pulmonary edema induced by detergent aerosol. J Appl Physiol 1985;58:129–136.
14. Bongard FS, Matthay MA, Mackensie RC, et al. Morphologic and physiologic correlates of increased extravascular lung water. Surgery 1984;96:395–403.
15. Gee MH, Spath JA. The dynamics of lung fluid filtration system in dogs with edema. Circ Res 1980;46:796–801.
16. Vreim CF, Snashall PD, Demling RH, et al. Lung lymph and free interstitial fluid protein composition in sheep with edema. J Appl Physiol 1976;230:1650–1653.
17. Vreim CF, Staub NC. Protein composition of lung fluids in acute alloxan edema in dogs. Am J Physiol 1976;230:376–379.
18. Fein AM, Goldberg SK, Walkenstein MD, et al. Is pulmonary artery catheterization necessary for the diagnosis of pulmonary edema? Am Rev Respir Dis 1984;129:1006–1009.
19. Matthay MA, Eschenbacher WC, Goetzl EJ. Elevated concentrations of leukotriene D_4 in pulmonary edema fluid of patients with the adult respiratory distress syndrome. J Clin Immunol 1984;4:479–483.
20. Aberle D, Wiener-Kronish JP, Webb R, et al. The diagnosis of hydrostatic versus increased permeability pulmonary edema based on chest radiographic criteria in critically ill patients. Radiology 1988;168:73–79.
21. Wiener-Kronish JP, Matthay MA. Pleural effusions are associated with hydrostatic and increased permeability pulmonary edema. Chest 1988;93:852–858.
22. Folkesson HG, Matthay MA, Hebert CA, et al. Acid aspiration induced lung injury in rabbits is mediated by interleukin-8 dependent mechanisms. J Clin Invest 1995;96:107–116.
23. Ohkuda K, Nakahara K, Binder A, et al. Venous air emboli in sheep: Reversible increase in lung vascular permeability. J Appl Physiol 1981;51:887–894.
24. Heflin AC, Brigham KL. Prevention by granulocyte depletion of increased vascular permeablity of sheep lung following endotoxemia. J Clin Invest 1981;68:1253–1260.
25. Landolt CC, Matthay MA, Albertine KH, et al. Overperfusion, hypoxia, and increased pressure caused only by hydrostatic pulmonary edema in anesthetized sheep. Circ Res 1983;52:335–341.
26. Gibbon JH Jr, Gibbon MH. Experimental pulmonary edema following lobectomy and plasma infusion. Surgery 1942;12:694–704.
27. Hultgren HN. High altitude pulmonary edema. In: Staub NC (ed). Lung Water and Solute Exchange. New York, Dekker, 1978, pp. 437–469.
28. Bachofen H, Schurch S, Michel RP, et al. Experimental hydrostatic pulmonary edema in rabbit lungs: Morphology. Am Rev Respir Dis 1993;147:989–996.
29. Bachofen H, Schurch S, Michel RP, et al. Experimental hydrostatic pulmonary edema in rabbit lungs: Barrier lesions. Am Rev Respir Dis 1993;147:997–1004.
30. West JB, Tsukimoto K, Mathieu-Costello O, et al. Stress failure in pulmonary capillaries. J Appl Physiol 1991;70:1731–1742.
31. Fu X, Costello ML, Tsukimoto K, et al. High lung volume increases stress failure in pulmonary capillaries. J Appl Physiol 1992;73:123–133.
32. West JB, Mathieu CO. High altitude pulmonary edema is caused by stress failure of pulmonary capillaries. Int J Sports Med S54, 1992.
33. Bartsch P, Maggiorini M, Ritter M, et al. Prevention of high-altitude pulmonary edema by nifedipine. N Engl J Med 1991;325:1284.

34. Colice GL, Matthay MA, Bass E, et al. Neurogenic pulmonary edema. Am Rev Respir Dis 1984;5:43–50.
35. Smith WS. The clinical incidence of hydrostatic versus increased permeability as the mechanism for neurogenic pulmonary edema. Am J Respir Crit Care Med, 1994.
36. Prewitt RM, McCarthy J, McCarthy LDH. Treatment of acute low pressure pulmonary edema in dogs. J Clin Invest 1981;67:409–418.
37. Matthay MA, Broaddus VC. Fluid and hemodynamic management in acute lung injury. Sem Resp Med 1994;15:271–288.
38. Unger KM, Shibel EM, Moser KM. Detection of left ventricular failure in patients with the adult respiratory distress syndrome. Chest 1975;67:8–13.
39. Cohen AB, Steven MD, Miller EJ, et al. Neutrophil-activating peptide-2 in patients with pulmonary edema from congestive heart failure or ARDS. Am J Physiol 1993;264:L490–L495.
40. Matthay MA, Landolt CC, Staub NC. Differential liquid and protein clearance from the alveoli of anesthetized sheep. J Appl Physiol 1982;53:96–104.
41. Matthay MA, Berthiaume Y, Staub NC. Long-term clearance of liquid and protein from the lungs of unanesthetized sheep. J Appl Physiol 1985;59:928–934.
42. Berthiaume Y, Broaddus VC, Gropper MA, et al. Alveolar liquid and protein clearance from normal dog lungs. J Appl Physiol 1988;65:585–593.
43. Matthay MA, Wiener-Kronish JP. Intact epithelial barrier function is critical for the resolution of alveolar edema in humans. Am Rev Respir Dis 1990;142:1250–1257.
44. Sakuma T, Pittet JF, Jayr C, et al. Alveolar liquid and protein clearance in the absence of blood flow or ventilation in sheep. J Appl Physiol 1993;74:176–185.
45. Matthay MA. Resolution of pulmonary edema: Mechanisms of liquid, protein, and cellular clearance from the lung. Clin Chest Med 1985;6:521–545.
46. Smedira N, Gates L, Hastings R, et al. Alveolar and lung liquid clearance in anesthetized rabbits. J Appl Physiol 1991;70:1827–1835.
47. Mason RJ, William MC, Widdecombe JH, et al. Transepithelial transport by pulmonary alveolar type II cells in primary culture. Proc Natl Acad Sci USA 1982;79:6033–6037.
48. Goodman BE, Crandall ED. Dome formation in primary cultured monolayers of alveolar epithelial cells. Am J Physiol 1982;243:C96–C100.
49. Cheek K, Kim KJ, Crandall ED. Tight monolayers of rat alveolar epithelial cells: Bioelectric properties and active sodium transport. Am J Physiol 1989;256:C688–C693.
50. Saumon G, Basset G. Electrolyte and fluid transport across the mature alveolar epithelium. J Appl Physiol 1993;74:1–15.
51. Matalon S. Mechanisms and regulation of ion transport in adult mammalian alveolar type II pneumocytes. Am J Physiol 1991;261:C727–C738.
52. Verkman AS. Water channels in cell membranes. Ann Rev Physiol 1992;54:97–108.
53. Folkesson HG, Matthay MA, Hasegawa H, et al. Transcellular water transport in lung alveolar epithelium through mercurial-sensitive water channels. Proc Natl Acad Sci USA 1994;91:4970–4974.
54. Berthiaume Y, Staub NC, Matthay MA. Beta-adrenergic agonists increase lung liquid clearance in anesthetized sheep. J Clin Invest 1987;79:335–343.
55. Jayr C, Garat C, Meignan C, et al. Alveolar liquid and protein clearance in anesthetized, ventilated rats. J Appl Physiol 1994;76(6):2636–2642.

56. Goodman BE, Fleischer RS, Crandall ED. Evidence for active Na+ transport by cultured monolayers of pulmonary alveolar epithelial cells. Am J Physiol 1983;245:C78–C83.
57. Crandall E, Heming RA, Palombo RL, et al. Effects of terbutaline on sodium transport in isolated perfused rat lung. J Appl Physiol 1986;60:289–294.
58. Sakuma OG, Nakada T, Nishimura T, et al. Alveolar fluid clearance in the resected human lung. Am J Resp Crit Care Med 1994;150:305–310.
59. Berthiaume Y, Albertine KH, Grady M, et al. Protein clearance from the air spaces and lungs of unanesthetized sheep over 144 h. J Appl Physiol 1989;67: 1887–1897.
60. Hastings RH, Grady M, Sakuma T, et al. Clearance of different-sized proteins from the alveolar space in humans and rabbits. J Appl Physiol 1992;73: 1310–1316.
61. Wiener-Kronish JP, Albertine KH, Matthay MA. Differential responses of the endothelial and epithelial barriers of the lung in sheep to Escherichia coli endotoxin. J Clin Invest 1991;88:864–875.
62. Wiener-Kronish JP, Broaddus VC, Albertine KH, et al. Relationship of pleural effusions to increased permeability pulmonary edema in anesthetized sheep. J Clin Invest 1988;82:1422–1429.
63. Cohen DS, Matthay MA, Cogan MG, et al. Acute lung injury associated with salt water drowning: New insights. Am Rev Respir Dis 1992;146:794–796.
64. Bachofen M, Weibel ER. Alterations of the gas exchange apparatus in adult respiratory insufficiency associated with septicemia. Am Rev Respir Dis 1977;116: 589–615.
65. Adamson IY, Bowden DH. The type II cell as progenitor of alveolar epithelial regeneration: A cytodynamic study in mice after exposure to oxygen. Lab Invest 1974;30:35–42.
66. Barrandon Y, Green H. Cell migration is essential for sustained growth of keratinocytes colonies: The role of TGF-a and EGF. Cell 1987;50:1131–1137.
67. Coomber BL, Gotlieb AI. In vitro endothelial wound repair. Arteriosclerosis 1990;10:215–222.
68. Kheradmand F, Folkesson HG, Shum L, et al. Transforming growth factor-a (TGF-a) enhances alveolar epithelial cell repair in a new *in vitro* model. AJP Lung Cellular and Molecular Physiology 1994;267:728.
69. Madtes DK, Raines EW, Sakariassen KS, et al. Induction of transforming growth factor -a in activated human alveolar macrophages. Cell 1988;53:285–293.
70. Strandjord TP, Clark JG, Hodson WA, et al. Expression of transforming growth factor-a in mid-gestation human fetal lung. Am J Resp Cell Mol Biol 1993;8: 266–272.
71. Raaberg L, Nexo E, Buckley S, et al. Epidermal growth factor transcription, translation and signal transduction by rat type II pneumocytes in culture. Am J Resp Cell Mol Biol 1992;6:44–49.
72. Matthay MA. Fibrosing alveolitis in the adult respiratory distress syndrome. Ann Intern Med 1995;122:65–66.

Chapter 3

Mechanism of Blood Flow During Cardiopulmonary Resuscitation

Donald L. Yakel Jr., M.D.,
Richard A. Podolin, M.D.

Cardiopulmonary resuscitation (CPR) provides the clearest and most dramatic example of cardiothoracic interaction. A force applied externally to the thorax is relied upon to provide the entire blood flow and organ perfusion necessary to sustain life until definitive therapy can be instituted. Successful CPR, that is, adequate ventilation and exploitation of cardiothoracic interaction, may result in a return to full and normal life. Failure of cardiothoracic interaction at this crucial junction, however, results in death within minutes.

The principles of CPR are simple enough to be taught to children, and the practice can be readily mastered by those with no medical or scientific background. Yet the physiology that underlies this unique intervention remains unclear. At least two theories have been proposed and it is likely that they are both, in part, correct. In this chapter we will discuss our understanding of cardiothoracic interaction as it applies in this unique and critical application.

History

The earliest reference to resuscitation is in Egyptian mythology. Isis, the healing goddess, breathes into her husband Osirio's mouth, restoring

From: Cosentino AM, Martin RJ (eds.): Cardiothoracic Interrelationships in Clinical Practice. © Futura Publishing Co., Inc., Armonk, NY, 1997.

him to life.[1] In 1543, Vasalius[2] ventilated a pig using a reed tube, and was able to observe the motion of the heart, lungs, and arteries in the opened chest. In 1667 Robert Hooke,[3] an English surgeon, ventilated a dog for more than 1 hour and proved the need for "fresh" air, rather than just motion of the lungs.

The modern concepts of CPR were established by Kouwenhoeven et al.[4] They demonstrated in a dog model that closed chest cardiac message allowed adequate circulation to be maintained for up to 30 minutes. They also reported four successful episodes of human resuscitation using rhythmical closed chest compression. The utility of closed chest resuscitation was soon confirmed by other investigators.[5,6] Kouwenhoeven et al.[4] hypothesized that forward blood flow during external chest compression occurred primarily as the result of compression of the ventricles between the sternum and spine. The motion and competence of the cardiac valves were presumed to be normal. This supposition was soon challenged. McKenzie et al.[7,8] used arterial and venous catheters to measure pressure and cardiac output in patients undergoing closed chest resuscitation. They demonstrated that right atrial and aortic root pressures were elevated equally during compression. They argued that external chest compression caused a generalized increase in intrathoracic pressure. This was supported by Criley et al.[9] who reported eight patients undergoing coronary angiography who were successfully resuscitated from ventricular fibrillation. They found that these patients could be kept conscious and alert for up to 39 seconds by following instructions to cough every 1–3 seconds. The mean aortic systolic pressure induced by cough (139.7 mmHg) was significantly higher than the pressure produced by external cardiac message (60.7 mmHg). These observations lead others to hypothesize that a generalized increase in intrathoracic pressure produced a systolic rise in aortic pressure that was the engine of forward blood flow during cardiac arrest. At the time, however, Criley et al.[9] postulated that blood flow during cough was caused by "rhythmic cardiac compression," holding to prior views of Kouwenhoven et al.[4]

Theories

As introduced above, two general theories have been advanced to explain the ability of CPR to "pump" blood from the systemic venous circulation to the systemic arterial circulation. These are the thoracic pump theory and the cardiac pump theory.

The cardiac pump theory originally proposed by Kouwenhoven et al.,[4] postulates that central chest compression during artificial systole squeezes the heart between the sternum and the spine, causing ejection of blood. According to this theory, indirect cardiac compression generates higher pressure in the ventricles than elsewhere in the thorax. The atrioventricular valves close and the semilunar valves open. Blood is ejected into the aorta and great arteries, and a positive arteriovenous pressure difference is generated. In artificial diastole (release of direct chest compression), intracardiac pressure falls as ventricular compression is relieved. The atrioventricular valves open, the semilunar valves close, and the heart fills from the systemic venous reservoir.

The "Thoracic Pump" theory, in contrast, proposes that forward blood flow during chest compression results from a generalized increase in intrathoracic pressure relative to extrathoracic pressure. Displacement of the sternum, direct cardiac compression, and even motion of the cardiac valves are largely irrelevant. In essence, all blood containing structures within the thorax are considered to be elastic tubes or chambers that are susceptible to collapse by external pressure. Chest compression causes a global increase in pressure in all structures of the thorax, including the heart, lungs, and pulmonary vessels. The great systemic veins carrying blood to the heart are easily collapsible by a small transmural pressure, and the aorta and its major branches tend to resist collapse except at high transmural pressures. As intrathoracic pressure rises during chest compression, both forward and backward flow are possible. Backward flow is decreased or stopped via the action of functional or mechanical venous valves at the thoracic inlet and beyond. Forward flow occurs through the left heart, aorta, and the pulmonary vasculature as a passive conduit. Generation of sufficient pressure in the intrathoracic space to force blood forward requires that there must be no or minimal venting of pressure through the bronchial tree. At the point where the arteries exit the thorax and become extrathoracic, a pressure gradient is generated allowing for forward flow. Blood flow then occurs through the high resistance vessels of the aorta and great arteries towards the lower resistance of the peripheral arteries and arterioles. If intrathoracic pressure increases beyond the critical transmural pressure that will collapse an artery, then forward flow will decrease or halt. During artificial diastole, intrathoracic pressure is relieved, and effective venous return allows blood flow into the heart. It is presumed that the aortic valve must close to prevent back flow of blood from the arterial tree. Filling of the thoracic pump therefore is accomplished via release of stored blood in the venous bed into the right heart as intrathoracic pressure drops (essentially using the stored energy of venous capacitance).

The essential components of the cardiac pump theory and the thoracic pump theory are quite different, yet both are based on previously known physiologic properties inherent to heart-lung interaction. The cardiac pump theory presumes that the heart remains an important component of the "pumping" system. Deformation of the left ventricular chamber is the major determinant of system pressure. The direction that this pressure is dissipated (blood flow) is directed just as it would be in a normal heart/ lung system, by the opening and closing of the aortic and mitral valves at the appropriate times. This causes forward blood flow during compression systole, and filling of the heart during release diastole. In contrast, the impetus for forward blood flow in the thoracic pump theory is provided by an increase in intrathoracic pressure. The left ventricular chamber and cardiac valves act only as a passive conduit through which blood flows unimpeded. An increase in intrathoracic pressure is equally distributed throughout every structure within the chest. This increase in pressure causes the compliant venous system to "collapse," preventing backward flow of blood into the venous system (this may also be assisted by functional venous valves at the thoracic inlet). The relative stiffness of the arterial tree keeps these passive conduits open, allowing forward flow of blood from the high pressure of the chest cavity into the peripheral arterial tree.

Experimental Studies: The Thoracic Pump Theory

The first direct evidence for a mechanism of forward blood flow during CPR was provided by Rudikoff et al.[10] who measured intrathoracic and intracardiac hemodynamics in dogs. During chest compression, pressures in the left ventricle, aorta, right atrium, pulmonary artery, and thoracic cavity (as measured by an esophageal balloon) were all essentially equal. These results favored the thoracic pump theory. There was relatively direct transmission of pressure from the aorta to the carotid artery with only a small pressure gradient between the two. In contrast, a large pressure gradient was demonstrated between the right atrium and the internal jugular vein and inferior vena cava. They hypothesized that this was the result of venous collapse, and cited as evidence the minimal retrograde venous flow during compression. Unequal transmission of pressures to the extrathoracic arterial and venous systems thus appeared to result from the collapse of the great veins at the thoracic inlet and patency of the great arteries at the thoracic outlet as intrathoracic pressures rose. Antegrade blood flow then occurred secondary to a peripheral arteriovenous pressure gradient. Increasing intrathoracic pressure during CPR by abdominal binding or inflation of the lungs produced reproducible and significant increases in aortic systolic pressure and carotid artery blood flow. The operation of a "venous valve" at the thoracic inlet was supported by the observation of a distinct pressure drop at the thoracic outlet in a patient who had a central venous catheter slowly removed from the right atrium to jugular vein during CPR.

Cineangiographic evidence from dog studies also supported the thoracic pump theory. Nieman et al.[11] demonstrated that ventricular volume did not decrease during closed chest compressions. Moreover, they demonstrated tricuspid valve insufficiency, an open mitral valve, an open aortic valve, and blood moving from the lung through the heart and into the aorta during chest compression. During release diastole, intrathoracic pressures fell toward zero with consequent venous flow into the right heart and lungs. The heart appeared to act only as a conduit allowing flow of blood from the elastic elements of the pulmonary circulation to the systemic circulation. These authors also felt that it was an elevation of pleural pressure and effective valves within the venous system that forced forward blood flow. They also presented angiographic evidence for a functional venous valve at the thoracic outlet, which could help to maintain an intrathoracic to extrathoracic venous pressure gradient. A modest gradient was shown to develop between the aorta and right atrium accounting for coronary artery blood flow. Further studies revealed that these findings could be confirmed in both large and small animals,[12] suggesting that chest configuration was not a key determinant of which theory was in effect.

Echocardiographic studies in humans during closed chest CPR have confirmed the angiographic findings in animal models.[13] The mitral and aortic valves did not close during release of chest pressure, but moved farther apart during "deep" chest compression. There was no demonstrable change in left ventricular size or shape, although the precision of these measurements was limited.

Halperin et al.[14] used a mathematical model of the cardiovascular system to predict changes in perfusion pressure and flow for changes in compression rate, compression duration, and applied force. Other models have predicted similar effects.[15,16] The model predicts that blood flow due to intrathoracic pressure fluctuations should be insensitive to compression rate but dependent on applied force and compression duration. Flow due to direct cardiac compression, in contrast, should vary with compression rate and force but be insensitive to compression duration above a threshold. Measurements in large mongrel dogs supported the thoracic pump model. Flow was significantly increased when the duration of compression was prolonged from 14% to 46% of cycle length at a constant rate and peak sternal force. Flow was unchanged by an increase in compression rate at constant compression duration.

Vest CPR was also found to cause a rise in intrathoracic pressure without significant sternal displacement, and produced myocardial perfusion pressures similar to those produced by conventional external chest CPR. These results provided strong support for the thoracic pump theory of CPR. The thoracic pump theory is also supported by the efficacy of "Vest CPR" in which chest compression is provided by the sudden rapid inflation of a pneumatic jacket. This has been shown to cause a rise in intrathoracic pressure without significant sternal displacement.[17–19]

Experimental Studies: The Cardiac Pump Theory

Since Kouwenhoven et al.[4] proposed the cardiac pump theory, a considerable body of supporting evidence has accumulated.[17–21] In contrast to large dog (>20-kg size) experiments, small dog (<10 kg) studies have documented left ventricular compression with closed chest cardiac resuscitation.[14,23] A 25% decrease in echocardiographic left ventricular area during compression systole has also been demonstrated in 20- to 30-kg minipigs.[20,23] Maier et al.[18] found vigorous chest compression in small animals (and only rarely with large dogs) produced intrathoracic vascular pressures that were much higher than intrapleural pressures. The excess rise in vascular pressures was likely the result of compression of the heart. Increasing the force of compression increased stroke volume up to a peak intrathoracic pressure of 20 mmHg. At higher pressures, stroke volume remained constant or declined. Ejection appeared to result primarily from direct transmission of compressive force to the heart since both peak cardiac and vascular pressures and the change in these pressures were consistently two to four times greater than intrathoracic pressures. Echocardiographic studies[19,20] have indicated that some degree of direct cardiac compression occurs in a quarter to a third of adult human patients during maximal compression. Together these studies suggest that the efficiency of the cardiac pump mechanism in CPR may be highly dependent on the conformation of the thoracic cage.

Echocardiographic studies in moderate sized dogs have demonstrated phasic movement of the cardiac valves, indicating phasic intracardiac pressure gradients. This result would be predicted from the cardiac pump theory. Using two-dimensional echocardiography, Feneley et al.[19] reported that the aortic valve opened with chest compression and closed with release. The mitral and tricuspid valves closed with compression and opened with release. With the onset of brief, high impulse chest compression, the mitral valve closed rapidly and the left ventricle was deformed whether compressions were applied to the sternum or the left chest mid-wall. The mitral valve reopened with release of each compression. The tricuspid and pulmonary valves also closed with compression and opened with release. Left atrial echocardiographic contrast injections confirmed the absence of anterograde transmitral blood flow during high impulse compression and its presence during release. Failure of mitral valve leaflet approximation during chest compression occurred only when a very low-velocity, prolonged (low impulse) compression technique was used.

Simultaneous recordings of the left ventricular and left atrial pressures during high impulse sternal compressions demonstrated peak and mean left ventriculoatrial pressure gradients of 39 and 14 mmHg, respectively. These pressure gradients declined with less aggressive chest compression. These observations in moderate sized dogs, subsequently replicated in 20- to 30-kg swine,[20,23] support direct cardiac compression as a mechanism of forward blood flow during CPR in all but low impulse chest compression modes. These findings were in direct contrast to the observations in large dogs made by Halperin[26] reported just 1 year earlier. Thus, both thoracic conformation and compression technique may determine the relative contribution of the cardiac pump.

Hackl et al.[27] performed CPR on anesthetized pigs using three different compressive forces delivered by mechanical means. Compressive forces of 200, 350, and 500 Newton (N) resulted in a decrease in anterior-posterior chest dimension of 15%, 20%, and 25%, respectively. During CPR systole with a compressive force of 200 N, the mitral valve closed in 16% of CPR cycles. At 350 N the mitral valve closed in 68% of cycles, and at 500 N it closed in 95% of cycles. These higher mitral valve closure rates were associated with significantly higher systolic cerebral perfusion pressures, diastolic myocardial perfusion pressures, and cardiac output. This study, like that of Feneley et al.,[19] strongly suggests that both thoracic and cardiac pumps function, but under different compressive forces. The thoracic pump may be more important with lower compressive forces, and the cardiac pump more responsible for the greatly augmented flow at higher applied pressures.

Interestingly, Deshmukh et al.[25] found valve motion during "compression systole" only in animals that were eventually resuscitated. Decreases in left ventricular dimensions, and transvalvular pressure gradients were no longer in evidence after 5 minutes of precordial compression in non-resuscitated animals. This may be one reason that valve motion and chamber deformation were not consistently found in some human studies.[22,28] In the minipig model, an aortic to right atrial pressure gradient of >20 mmHg was required for successful resuscitation. The persistence of valve function, chamber compression, and pressure gradients during precordial compression was predictive of successful resuscitation. The absence of these factors similarly predicted a failure of resuscitation. These observations provide strong evidence that the cardiac pump mechanism is necessary if CPR is to be successful. They also may explain the inconsistent findings of earlier studies in which the outcome of resuscitation was not reported.[22,28]

Transesophageal echocardiography (TEE) affords visualization of the intracardiac structures with greater clarity and resolution than standard transthoracic techniques. TEE in humans during CPR has generally confirmed direct compression of the right and left ventricles, aortic valve opening, and mitral valve closure during compression systole.[30,31] The observation of atrioventricular regurgitation during compression systole in some patients indicates a positive ventricular to atrial pressure gradient.[31] In a few patients, however, CPR did not produce significant ventricular compression[32] or mitral valve closure.[30]

New Techniques

Standard CPR produces at most 30% of the normal resting cardiac output.[17] Coronary perfusion pressure is often less than the 15- to 30-mmHg gradient necessary to permit the return of spontaneous circulation from more than momentary cardiac arrest.[17,18] Therefore modifications have been promoted to increase perfusion during CPR. These modifications, in general, tighten the coupling of cardiothoracic interaction. Factors that limit blood flow during CPR include those that limit filling and those that limit emptying of the pumping chamber. Filling of the heart during artificial diastole depends on the pressure difference between the great veins and right ventricle (cardiac pump theory) or between the great veins and the intrathoracic vascular space (thoracic pump theory). Measures to increase this gradient that have been tried include: the application of negative airway pressure during diastole; fluid loading; abdominal binding; and leg elevation.

Emptying of the cardiac pump is proportional to the pressure gradient between the left ventricle and the systemic arterial bed (cardiac pump theory) or between the intrathoracic and extrathoracic arterial vascular beds (thoracic pump theory), and inversely proportional to the peripheral resistance. Methods to increase this pressure difference (emptying) include increasing sternal displacement, preventing displacement of the heart to the side (perhaps by simultaneous lung inflation and chest compression), and decreasing outflow resistance with selective arteriolar dilating agents (although these do not increase the likelihood of survival).

Static abdominal binding has been used to inhibit diastolic runoff from the thoracic aorta to non-vital vascular beds.[24,29,35] This, in turn, raises the aortic-to-right atrial pressure gradient driving perfusion of the heart and brain. A hemodynamic benefit for several minutes or more has been documented, but there have been serious concerns about the possibility of liver damage and intraperitoneal hemorrhage.

One attractive means of securing the hemodynamic benefits of abdominal pressurization, while maintaining a low risk of visceral trauma, is to compress the abdomen only during the diastolic phase of chest compression. Interposed abdominal compression CPR (IAC CPR) may avoid entrapment of the liver between the sternum and the spine as the chest compression pushes the liver caudally. These techniques have been discussed in detail elsewhere.[33]

Contact compression occurs to the extent that the localized external force applied to the abdominal wall is directly transmitted through intervening tissues to the underlying structures such as the aorta and great veins. Hydrostatic compression, in contrast, occurs to the extent that a generalized rise in intraabdominal pressure is created and transmitted uniformly to all sides of intraabdominal structures. Two hemodynamic mechanisms may mediate the effect of abdominal compression. First, contact compression of the abdominal aorta during chest recoil squeezes blood retrograde toward the heart and brain similar to the diastolic augmentation that occurs with an intraaortic balloon pump. In essence, an abdominal pump is added to the thoracic and/or cardiac pump. Unlike the intraaortic balloon pump, abdominal compression should induce pressure pulses in both arteries and veins. In order to improve coronary blood flow by contact compression, the augmentation of central aortic pressure must be greater than the increase in central venous pressure. This could indeed occur due to the greater capacitance of the venous system. Second, both hydrostatic and contact compression in IAC CPR may "prime" the thoracic or cardiac pump by increasing intrathoracic blood volume prior to compression systole. Pearson and Redding[19] noted in animal models of cardiac arrest over two decades ago that application of interventions that increase extrathoracic vascular resistance, such as alpha adrenergic drugs or mechanical abdominal binding, produced a positive influence on blood flow indices. Moreover, a given systemic arteriovenous pressure difference superimposed on the higher venous pressure pedestal produced by IAC may more easily overcome capillary closing pressure. IAC CPR raises systolic and diastolic arterial pressure and improves cardiac output, arteriovenous pressure difference, and carotid blood flow in both animal and human studies,[36–44] although a survival benefit has not been demonstrated.[43,44] Thus, raising venous pressure, if it can be done without compromising the arteriovenous pressure, may itself improve tissue perfusion.

Simultaneous pressure applied to the chest and abdomen may generate higher thoracic aortic pressures than IAC.[45] The effects of synchronized compression on flow dynamics and, ultimately, survival is uncertain. Simultaneous cyclical high pressure ventilation and closed chest compression increased flow to the heart and brain in dogs[33] when compared to standard CPR. This has had limited use in clinical practice, however, because of the need for endotracheal intubation and complex mechanical devices. Halperin et al.[18] used a pneumatically cycled vest placed around the thorax (Vest CPR). Vest CPR utilizes a pneumatic jacket to cyclically increase intrathoracic pressure. This might be expected to augment a thoracic pump more efficiently than a cardiac pump but experimental confirmation of this is lacking. In dog studies in which vest CPR has been compared to standard CPR, vest CPR improves myocardial and cerebral blood flow with less injury to the ribs and liver.[18] The higher vest pressures associated with an increase in blood flow over that seen in standard CPR were associated with a significant increase in organ trauma from the technique. Studies in humans have also demonstrated increases in peak aortic systolic pressure and myocardial perfusion pressure.[20,21] In one small study, while vest CPR improved immediate recovery rate, none of the resuscitated patients survived to hospital discharge.[21] As in other studies, a hemodynamic benefit for vest CPR was shown but no clear survival benefit was documented.

Active compression/decompression CPR (ACD CPR) has received considerable attention since the report of a successful resuscitation using a simple household plunger.[23] A more efficient device, based on the same principle, has since been developed.[46] In this variation on standard CPR a suction cup applied to the chest wall is used to actively retract the anterior chest during decompression diastole as well as to compress the chest during "systole." Active diastolic retraction of the chest wall could improve the hemodynamic performance of either the thoracic or cardiac pump. The negative intrathoracic pressure generated would increase venous return, "priming" the thoracic and cardiac pumps in much the same way as abdominal compression. In addition, negative intrapleural pressure would promote passive left ventricular filling by increasing the transmural pressure difference (intracardiac minus pleural) expanding the ventricle.

In animal and human studies ACD CPR improves diastolic left ventricular filling and raises systolic arterial pressure, stroke volume, and cardiac output.[46–48] In clinical studies initial resuscitation rates have been double that of standard CPR.[47,48] A trend toward improved survival to hospital discharge has also been found.[47,48] Overall survival rates remain low, however, attesting to the severity of the underlying conditions that precipitate cardiopulmonary arrest.

Summary

When active cardiac contraction is interrupted, cardiothoracic interaction can be exploited to sustain life through the techniques of CPR. Two theories have emerged to explain the mechanisms by which external thoracic compression produces intravascular circulation. The thoracic pump theory suggests that a generalized increase in intrathoracic pressure is transmitted more readily to the great arteries than to the extrathoracic veins. The resultant arteriovenous pressure gradient drives blood flow. The heart itself functions as a passive conduit like other intrathoracic vascular structures. The cardiac pump theory, in contrast, proposes that the force of external chest compression is transmitted more directly to the ventricles, raising the pressures in these chambers in a manner analogous to active contraction.

Current evidence suggests that both mechanisms may be operational. The predominance of one mechanism over the other may depend upon the technique of compression. The enhancement of flow that results from recruitment of the cardiac pump may be a requirement for successful resuscitation, however, when manual chest compression is performed.

New techniques have emerged that tighten the coupling between external thoracic compression and blood flow. While these advancements offer hope for improved survival, their efficacy is limited by the severity of the underlying medical conditions that precipitate cardiopulmonary arrest.

References

1. Lyons AS, Petrucelli RJ. Medicine: An Illustrated History. New York, Abrams, 1976.
2. Thangam S, Weil MH, Rackow EC. Cardiopulmonary resuscitation: A historical review. Acute Care 1986;12:63–94.
3. Hooke R. External cardiac massage. Philos Trans R Soc Lond 1667;2:539–540.
4. Kouwenhoven WB, Jude JR, Knickerbocker GG. Closed chest cardiac massage. JAMA 1960;173:1064–1067.
5. Baringer JR, Salzman EW, Jones WA, et al. N Engl J Med 1961;265:62.
6. Jude JR, Kouwenhoven WB, Knickerbocker GG. A new approach to cardiac resuscitation. Am Surg 1961;154:311–319.
7. Weale FE, Rothwell-Jackson RL. The efficiency of cardiac message. Lancet 1961;1:990.
8. MacKenzie GJ, Taylor SH, McDonald AH, et al. Hemodynamic effects of external cardiac compression. Lancet 1990;1:1342–1345.
9. Criley JM, Blaufuss AH, Kissel GL. Cough induced cardiac compression-self administered form of cardiopulmonary resuscitation. JAMA 1976;236:1246–1250.
10. Rudikoff MT, Maughan WL, Effron M, et al. Mechanisms of blood flow during cardiopulmonary resuscitation. Circulation 1980;61:345–353.
11. Niemann JT, Rasbrough JP, Hausknecht M, et al. Pressure synchronized cineangiography during experimental cardiopulmonary resuscitation. Circulation 1981;64:985–991.
12. Fisher J, Vaghaiwalle F, Tsitlike JE. Determinants and clinical significance of jugular venous valve competence. Circulation 1982;65:1988.
13. Werner JA, Greene HL, Janko CL, et al. Visualization of cardiac valve motion in man during external chest compression using 2D echocardiography, implications regarding the mechanism of blood flow. Circulation 1981;63:1417–1421.
14. Halperin HR, Tsitlike JE, Guerci AD, et al. Determinants of blood flow to vital organs during cardiopulmonary resuscitation in dogs. Circulation 1986;73: 539–550.

15. Babbs C, Weaver JC, Ralston S, et al. Cardiac, thoracic, and abdominal pump mechanisms in cardiopulmonary resuscitation: Studies in an electrical model of the circulation. Am J Emerg Med 1984;2:299.
16. Beyar R, Kishon Y, Sideman S, et al. Computer studies of systemic and regional blood flow mechanisms during cardiopulmonary resuscitation. Med Biol Eng Comp 1984;22:499.
17. Babbs CF. New versus old theories of blood flow during cardiopulmonary resuscitation. Crit Care Med 1980;8:191–196.
18. Halperin HR, Guerci AD, Chandra N. Vest inflation without simultaneous ventilation during cardiac arrest in dogs: Improved survival from prolonged cardiopulmonary resuscitation. Circulation 1986;74:1407–1415.
19. Feneley MP, Maier GW, Gaynor JW, et al. Sequence of mitral valve motion and transmitral blood flow during manual cardiopulmonary resuscitation in dogs. Circulation 1987;76:363–375.
20. Swenson RD, Weaver WD, Niskanen RA. Hemodynamics in humans during conventional and experimental methods of cardiopulmonary resuscitation. Circulation 1988;78:630–639.
21. Halperin HR, Tsitlike JE, Gelfand M, et al. A preliminary study of cardiopulmonary resuscitation by circumferential compression of the chest with use of pneumatic vest. N Engl J Med 1993;329:762–768.
22. Rich S, Wix HL, Shapiro EP. Clinical assessment of heart chamber size and valve motion during cardiopulmonary resuscitation by two-dimensional echocardiography. Am Heart J 1981;102:368–373.
23. Birch LH, Kenney LJ, Doornbos F, et al. A study of external cardiac compression. Mich State Med Soc J 1962;61:1346–1352.
24. Redding JS. Abdominal compression in cardiopulmonary resuscitation. Anesth Analg 1971;50:668–675.
25. Desmukh HG, Weil MH, Chalipathirao VG, et al. Mechanism of blood flow generated by precordial compression during CPR. Chest 1971;95:1092–1099.
26. Deshmukh HG, Weil MH, Rackow EC, et al. Echocardiographic observations during cardiopulmonary resuscitation: A preliminary report. Crit Care Med 1989;13:904–906.
27. Hackl WS, Simon P, Mouritz W, et al. Echocardiographic assessment of mitral valve function during mechanical cardiopulmonary resuscitation in pigs. Anesth Analg 1990;70:350–356.
28. Werner JA, Greene HL, Janko CL, et al. Visualization of cardiac valve motion in man during external chest compression using two-dimensional echocardiography: Implications regarding the mechanism of blood flow. Circulation 1981;63:1417–1421.
29. Harris LC, Kirinili B, Safar P. Augmentation of artificial circulation during cardiopulmonary resuscitation. Anesthesiology 1967;28:730–734.
30. Porter TR, Ornato TP, Guard CS, et al. Transesophageal echocardiography to assess mitral valve function and flow during cardiopulmonary resuscitation. Am J Cardiol 1992;70:1056–1060.
31. Redberg RF, Tucker KJ, Cohen TJ, et al. Physiology of blood flow during cardiopulmonary resuscitation: A transesophageal echocardiographic study. Circulation 1993;88:534–542.
32. Clements FM, DeBruijn NP, Kisslo JA. Transesophageal echocardiographic observations in a patient undergoing closed-chest massage. Anesthesiology 1988;64:826–828.

33. Babbs CF, Sack JB, Kern KB. Interposed abdominal compression as an adjunct to cardiopulmonary resuscitation. Am Heart J 1994;127:412–421.
34. Maier GW, Tyson GS, Oben CO. The physiology of external cardiac massage: High impulse cardiopulmonary resuscitation. Circulation 1984;70:86–101.
35. Chandra N, Snyder LD, Weisfeldt ML. Abdominal binding during cardiopulmonary resuscitation in man. JAMA 1981;246:351–353.
36. Ralston SH, Babbs CF, Niebauer MJ. Cardiopulmonary resuscitation with interposed manual compression in dogs. Anesth Analg 1982;61:645–651.
37. Voorhees WD, Babbs CF, Niebauer MJ. Improved oxygen delivery during cardiopulmonary resuscitation with interposed abdominal compressions. Ann Emerg Med 1983;12:128–135.
38. Einagle V, Bertrand F, Wise RA, et al. Interposed abdominal compressions and carotid blood flow during cardiopulmonary resuscitation: Support for a thoracoabdominal unit. Chest 1988;93:1206–1212.
39. Coletti RH, Kaskel PS, Cohen SR, et al. Abdominal counterpulsation (AC)-A new concept in circulatory assistance. Trans Am Soc Artif Intern Organs 1982; 28:563–566.
40. Coletti RH, Kaskel PS, Gregman D. Abdominal counterpulsation during cardiopulmonary resuscitation: Effects of canine coronary and carotid blood flow. Circulation 1983;64(Suppl 2):226–231.
41. Lindner KH, Annefeld FW, Bowdler IM. Cardiopulmonary resuscitation with interposed abdominal compression after asphyxial or fibrillatory cardiac arrest in pigs. Anesthesiology 1990;72:675–681.
42. Berryman CR, Phillips GM. Interposed abdominal compression-CPR in human subjects. Ann Emerg Med 1984;13:226–229.
43. Sack JB, Kesselbrenner MB, Bregman D. Survival from in hospital cardiac arrest with interposed abdominal counterpulsation during cardiopulmonary resuscitation. JAMA 1992;267:379–385.
44. Mateer JR, Stueven HA, Thompson BM. Interposed abdominal compression CPR versus standard CPR in pre-hospital cardiopulmonary arrest: Preliminary results. (abstract) Am J Emerg Med 1984;2:354.
45. Barranco F, Lesmer A, Irles JA. Cardiopulmonary resuscitation with simultaneous chest and abdominal compression: Comparative study in humans. Resuscitation 1990;20:67–77.
46. Tucker KJ, Redburg RF, Schiller NB, et al. Active compression-decompression resuscitation: Analysis of transmitral flow and left ventricular volume by transesophageal echocardiography in humans. Cardiopulmonary Resusciation Working Group. J Am Coll Cardiol 1993;22:1485–1493.
47. Cohen TJ, Goldner BG, Maccaw PC, et al. A comparison of active compression-decompression cardiopulmonary resuscitation with standard cardiopulmonary resuscitation for cardiac arrest occurring in the hospital. N Engl J Med 1993; 329:1918–1921.
48. Tucker KJ, Galle F, Savitt MA, et al. Active compression-decompression resuscitation-effect on resuscitation success after in-hospital cardiac arrest. J Am Coll Cardiol 1994;24:201–209.

Chapter 4

Respiratory Considerations in Congestive Heart Failure:

Pathophysiology, Assessment, and Management

P. Anthony Haddad, M.D., Christopher A. Bailey, M.D., Barry A. Gray, M.D., Ph.D.

Although the heart and lungs share the thoracic cage and are intimately interconnected, it is common to think of these two systems as separate and independent, a misconception that has been perpetuated by the intense specialization that has occurred in medicine. Clinicians, however, who manage cardiorespiratory diseases have long identified the need to view these systems together with the recognition that alterations in one can produce simultaneous changes in the other. The care of a patient with cardiogenic pulmonary edema (CPE) brings to bear many of the intricate relationships between the two systems. The clinical descriptive term "cardiac asthma" for CPE further epitomizes this close association. Knowledge of the pathophysiology involved in this particular disease state provides insight into how pathological changes in the cardiac system impact on the pulmonary system to produce a characteristic clinical picture. The intent of this chapter, therefore, is to examine the pulmonary manifestations observed in cardiac failure. Specifically, we look at alterations in pulmonary mechanics and gas exchange in this clinical setting and the implications for diagnosis, management, and prognosis in these patients.

From: Cosentino AM, Martin RJ (eds.): Cardiothoracic Interrelationships in Clinical Practice. © Futura Publishing Co., Inc., Armonk, NY, 1997.

Evolution of Pulmonary Edema

To fully appreciate the changes that occur in pulmonary function as a consequence of CPE, a brief review of the stages involved in the evolution of pulmonary edema is essential. These stages are as follows:

Pulmonary Congestion

Pulmonary congestion is the stage in which there is an increase in pulmonary blood volume without an increase in extravascular lung water (EVLW).

Interstitial Edema

Interstitial edema is further divided into extra-alveolar and alveolar interstitial edema in which fluid accumulates first in the bronchovascular interstitium then spills over into the alveolar interstitium.[1]

Alveolar Edema

Progression to alveolar edema involves flooding of the alveoli with fluid that moves across the epithelial surface of an alveolus or its associated alveolar duct or respiratory bronchiole.[2] Microscopic studies indicate that during the development of alveolar edema, individual alveoli are either completely flooded or dry. Partially flooded alveoli are not found, but there may be small collections of liquid in the corners of some alveoli.[1]

These stages are obviously an oversimplification of the process of pulmonary edema formation in the setting of CPE. For example, recent work has suggested that the mechanism responsible for the formation of alveolar edema involves not only the fluid movement along a pressure gradient but also increased permeability.[3–5] Tsukimoto et al.[5] showed that high capillary hydrostatic pressures cause changes within the ultrastructure of the capillary walls producing disruptions within the endothelium and epithelium. Nevertheless, since each of the above stages have fairly distinctive changes in pulmonary function, the use of the above staging system fits our purposes and will be referred to often in the following discussion.

Pulmonary Mechanics

Restriction

The conventional wisdom has been to think of congestive heart failure (CHF) as producing restrictive pulmonary function.

Lung Volumes

Vital Capacity. One of the simplest and most practical measurements of changes in pulmonary mechanics is the vital capacity (VC). The literature is replete with clinical observations documenting a reduced VC in patients with CHF. The clinical relevance and prognostic value of this association was highlighted by the classic work of Peabody and Wentworth[6] in 1917. Patients with lower VCs had higher mortalities, more symptoms, and were less likely to be employed. In addition, changes in VC in a given patient mirrored his clinical status. Kannel[7] examined the efficacy of VC to detect impending heart failure and found that a persistently low VC or a recent fall in VC was associated with increased risk of decompensated heart failure. Similar observations of the VC as a sensitive parameter for changes in hemodynamic status following acute myocardial infarction (AMI) have also been made.[8–10] As illustrated in Figure 1, reduced VC can provide a noninvasive means to estimate the severity of left ventricular (LV) failure and changes in LV filling pressure.

Total Lung Capacity. Reduced total lung capacity (TLC) has been observed not only in frank pulmonary edema but also in situations characterized by pulmonary congestion or interstitial edema without alveolar edema.[10–13] The mechanisms of the reduction in TLC involve changes in lung compliance and changes in chest wall mechanics.

Functional Residual Capacity and Residual Volume. There is less general agreement about the changes in functional residual capacity (FRC) and residual volume in CHF. The earliest studies of residual air in patients with cardiac failure indicated that residual volume was decreased in the presence of decompensation, but the reduction of residual volume was not as striking as the reduction in VC.[14] Frank and coworkers[15] published measurements of FRC and residual volume in patients with CHF obtained by nitrogen washout in the supine position. Compared with normal values from other laboratories[16] the FRC averaged 62.6%±11.5% of predicted and the residual volume 76%±21.4% of predicted. Measurement of residual volume or

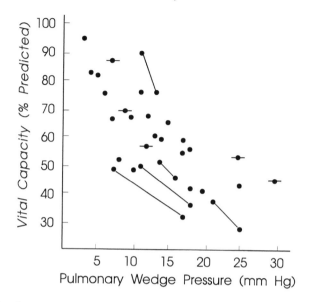

Figure 1. Simultaneous vital capacity and wedge pressure measurements in 29 patients with acute myocardial infarction during the first 4 days after hospital admission. Horizontal lines through points represent five patients in whom repeat measurements revealed changes of <3 mmHg in wedge pressure and <4% in vital capacity. Pairs of connected points represent five who experienced greater changes in wedge pressure and vital capacity.

FRC requires either body plethysmography or gas dilution methods. Patients with acute CHF are usually too ill for study in the body plethysmograph and in this group of acutely ill patients with AMI, gas dilution measurements indicate reduced FRC and residual volume with the reduction in volume paralleling the severity of abnormality in pulmonary hemodynamics.[10,17] In patients in whom AMI had been excluded, body plethysmography did not reveal consistent reductions in FRC and residual volume.[18] Whether this represents a fundamental difference between the acutely ill patient or merely a difference in methodology has not been established. Hales and Kazemi[9] found that residual volume may be increased slightly in uncomplicated and myocardial infarction, but with more pronounced pulmonary congestion and edema they found that residual volume is reduced. Light and George[18] found a substantial difference in residual volume obtained by plethysmography as compared with nitrogen washout in stable patients with CHF. In fact, residual volume as assessed by phlethysmography was 1.04 L greater than that measured by nitrogen washout. With further clinical improvement, this difference was reduced to 0.520 L. Such a discrepancy is well described in obstructive lung disease where there is uneven distribution of ventilation producing an underestimation of total gas volume with techniques such as nitrogen washout.[19]

In normal subjects, pulmonary vascular congestion produced by blood volume expansion or by the inflation of medical anti-shock trousers (MAST pants) produces acute and reversible decreases in FRC.[12,20] There are also observations in experimental animals that provide direct evidence for a reduction in FRC with pulmonary vascular engorgement.[21]

Lung Compliance

Decreased lung compliance has been correlated with reductions in TLC and VC with the greatest alterations in those patients with alveolar edema.[15,22] In comparison with pulmonary edema, vascular congestion without edema has only a small effect on lung compliance in healthy human subjects[23,24] or anesthetized dogs.[21] In dogs with edema, Noble et al.[25] demonstrated that the fall in lung compliance is directly proportional to increasing extravascular lung water. These observations highlight the fact that alveolar flooding is the main factor resulting in reduced compliance by simple replacement of alveolar volume with edema fluid as well as alteration of geometric and surface forces working to keep alveoli open.[26] Therefore, in acute pulmonary edema, the decrease in compliance is primarily a function of the number of alveoli with edema rather than changes in the elastic framework of the lung. In chronic CHF, however, lung elasticity may be altered with the development of peribronchial and alveolar interstitial fibrosis contributing to reduced compliance.[27,28]

Chest Wall Mechanics

Anatomic abnormalities such as pleural effusions, cardiomegaly, or ascites have a direct effect that reduces lung gas volume and increases pleural pressure. Increased pulmonary blood volume can also contribute to reduced lung gas volume. Partial mitral valve obstruction in dogs produces an immediate decrease in lung gas volume and increase in pleural pressure.[21] As a consequence of the increased pulmonary blood volume, there is increased chest wall volume, whereas lung gas volume is decreased. Similarly, in human subjects given acute volume expansion, the reduction in FRC reflects the increase in central blood volume.[12]

These changes in chest wall mechanics, with decreased lung gas volume and increased chest wall volume, are similar to those seen with pleural effusion or external pneumothorax, and may be partially responsible for the dyspnea of CHF. Estenne and colleagues[29] suggest that the mechanism for the relief of dyspnea after thoracentesis involved an improvement in the mechanical advantage of the inspiratory muscles as chest wall volume is decreased. After thoracentesis, they demonstrated that inspiratory pleural pressure values were significantly more negative at any comparable lung gas volume—a change that they attributed to a reduction in thoracic cage volume with subsequent improvement in inspiratory muscle mechanical advantage. It would follow that a reduction in congestion might also restore the respiratory muscles to a more advantageous position and improve strength and function.

Obstruction

Airway obstruction as a consequence of heart failure has been suggested by a variety of clinical and animal data.[18,30–34] Clinicians have been aware for years that patients with acute pulmonary edema may present with a picture consistent with asthma and hence the coining of the phrase "cardiac asthma." Plotz[31] first demonstrated reversible airway obstruction in patients with heart failure when he noted rapid improvement in vital capacity with epinephrine—an effect that he attributed to relief of bronchiolar spasm. Since Plotz's[31] study, there has been much work to define the mechanisms associated with airflow obstruction in this setting. It has become increasingly clear that the mechanism is multifactorial and dependent on the stage of pulmonary edema. Competition within the bronchovascular sheath, increased bronchial hyperresponsiveness, stimulation of vagal afferents, smooth muscle contraction, submucosal and bronchial wall edema have all been put forward as operative mechanisms.

Changes in Airway Resistance

There is little argument that once alveolar edema ensues there is an increase in both central and peripheral airways resistance. This has been demonstrated by many investigators.[25,26,35] The observations by Sharp et al.[26] are particularly noteworthy in regard to mechanism. In patients with alveolar edema, they found a threefold increase in airway resistance. Because of the extremely high airway resistance noted at the onset of inspiration, they inferred that bubbles in the edema froth may play a significant role in generating the changes in pulmonary mechanics.[26] Other contributing factors for increased airway resistance in this setting are suggested by observations in animals and humans studied in the earlier stages of pulmonary edema.

Animal Data. The early stages of pulmonary congestion and interstitial edema are characterized by increased airway resistance, but of much lesser degree than with alveolar edema. This is related to the fact that these stages are characterized by increases in peripheral airway resistance, which has been shown to account for <10% of the total airway resistance.[36] In dogs, Hogg et al.[33] demonstrated that elevation of left atrial pressure (P_{LA}) to 15 cm H_2O with subsequent return to baseline produced reversible increases in peripheral airway resistance especially at low lung volumes with no change in central airway resistance. Further elevation of P_{LA} to 30 cm H_2O produced larger and much less reversible changes in peripheral resistance. The authors concluded that the initial reversible phase was likely due to competition for space in the bronchovascular bundle caused by vascular congestion whereas the irreversible changes were related to interstitial and alveolar edema.

Mechanical Effects of Vascular Congestion and Edema. The conclusions of Hogg et al.[33] bring up the often quoted mechanism of compression of the small airways by interstitial edema to account for changes in airway resistance in these early stages.[33,37,38] This has been refuted, however, by Michel and associates[39] who demonstrated by morphometric analysis that airway areas and diameters did not decrease in dogs with hydrostatic pulmonary edema induced by volume overload. They concluded that interstitial edema was not responsible for changes in airway resistance and suggested that other mechanisms must be operative.

Neurogenic Reflex Effects. Reflexes mediated by the vagus nerve through a variety of afferent receptors represent an additional mechanism for increased airway resistance.[34,40,41] Chung and colleagues[42] presented radiographic evidence of decreased lung volume and airway caliber with the induction of pulmonary edema in dogs. Vagotomy, or vagal cooling, did not prevent the fall in lung volume, but the airway caliber was returned to the control value. Ishii and colleagues[34] defined three discrete stages in the development of hydrostatic pulmonary edema. The early stage was characterized by a prompt and significant increase in peripheral airway resistance that could be abolished by vagotomy. The second stage was characterized by a gradual increase in peripheral and central airway resistance not influenced by vagal reflexes. This stage was believed to result from peribronchial and endobronchial edema. The final stage, characterized by a rapid rise in both the central and peripheral airway resistance, was believed to result from alveolar flooding and bronchial froth with bubble formation.

In an effort to identify which vagal afferents may be involved and at what stage of pulmonary edema they are functional, Roberts and associates[41] studied activation of vagal afferents in dogs with either pulmonary congestion and edema or edema alone. They found that pulmonary congestion with edema results in stimulation of rapidly adapting receptors as well as bronchial and pulmonary C-fibers. Furthermore, edema without congestion still produced significant, albeit less intense, stimulation of the bronchial and pulmonary C-fibers. This is pertinent because stimulation of these receptors is known to cause bronchoconstriction and increase airway secretions.

Clinical Data. Numerous clinical studies have shown abnormalities in various parameters characteristic of small airways obstruction. For instance, with pacing-induced angina pectoris resulting in a sudden increase in left ventricular end-diastolic pressure (LVEDP) and pulmonary congestion, Pepine and Weiner[43] found significant reductions in specific airway conductance, which abruptly return to normal with resolution of angina. In acute myocardial infarction characterized by vascular engorgement and interstitial edema, there are modest increases in airway resistance as well as signs of small airway obstruction including the development of frequency dependence of resistance and an increased closing volume (CV).[8,44] Similar findings in regard to small airway dysfunction have been reported in subjects receiving rapid saline infusion.[11,20,45] These changes in the small airways have been related to clinical symptoms. For example, in the study by Pepine and Weiner,[43] anginal symptoms of dyspnea and chest tightness corresponded temporally with changes in airway conductance, suggesting a causal relationship. Collins et al.[46] found a significant relationship with dyspnea severity and length of symptoms and the ratio closing volume/vital capacity. Of note, no relationship was found between this ratio and vascular pressures.

As in animal studies, evidence for changes in airway resistance mediated by the vagus also exists in humans. Goeree et al.[20] showed that atropine, when given prior to saline infusion, prevented an increase in the slope of phase III nitrogen washout supporting the notion that the increase in small airways resistance is mediated by vagal reflex.

The observation that atropine reversed the fall in lung compliance associated with pulmonary vascular congestion produced by dextran infusion in normal human subjects is also of interest in terms of changes in smooth muscle tone mediated by the vagus.[12] In that study, Giuntini and coworkers[12] measured both static and dynamic lung compliance and noted a greater reduction in dynamic than static lung compliance with congestion and a greater increase in dynamic compliance with atropine after congestion. Although measured at points of zero airflow, changes in airway resistance leading to inhomogeneities in the distribution of ventilation can produce changes in dynamic compliance. The increase in static compliance produced by atropine in pulmonary vascular congestion, however, cannot be attributed to changes in airflow resistance. Nor can it be attributed to changes in vascular volume since neither central nor pulmonary blood volume decreased. In fact, the latter increased. The authors interpret the response to atropine in pulmonary vascular congestion as evidence that changes in parenchymal smooth muscle tone mediated by the vagus nerve contribute to the fall in compliance.

Obstructive Spirometry in Patients with Congestive Heart Failure

When VC is reduced, it is common practice to use the ratio of forced expiratory volume in 1 second (FEV_1) to forced vital capacity (FVC) to detect airflow obstruction. Reductions in the FEV_1/FVC ratio are believed to indicate airflow obstruction in more central airways. Using this measurement, there has been conflicting data in the literature in defining an obstructive defect in heart failure. Most studies[8,9,32] have shown that the reduction in FEV_1 is proportional to the reduction in VC implying primarily a restrictive process. In contrast, Light and George[18] reported serial pulmonary function measurements in 28 heart failure patients of whom 15 were nonsmokers. Acutely, 61% of the patients had a reduced FEV_1/FVC ratio including 67% of the nonsmokers. A reduced ratio persisted in 53% of the latter group in the follow-up period consistent with a mild obstructive defect at baseline.

Effect of Treatment. Support for obstruction as a major manifestation of acute heart failure can be demonstrated by the clinical response to therapy. Sharp et al.[47] observed a prompt decrease in airway resistance and increase in compliance after the intravenous administration of aminophylline to patients with pulmonary edema. Heyer[48] showed an acute increase in FVC with aminophylline in patients with cardiac asthma and Plotz[31] showed similar increases in FVC with the use of epinephrine in patients with CHF. These data add credence to the idea that FVC is reduced in large part as a consequence of obstruction and air trapping.

The response to treatment with an anticholinergic agent suggests that the role played by the vagal mechanisms depends on the severity of the pulmonary vascular congestion and edema. Rolla et al.[49] examined the response to inhaled ipratropium bromide both during the acute exacerbation of CHF, and after intensive therapy with diuretics, sodium restriction, vasodilators, and cardiac glycosides for 7–10 days. In the acute phase of the study, these patients had significant restrictive ventilatory impairment with TLC equal to 77% of predicted, but also an undeniable obstructive component with FEV_1/FVC equal to 0.61. At this point ipratropium produced significant bronchodilatation with a 20% increase in FEV_1. In the second phase of the study, when there had been marked clinical and radiographic improvement and TLC was 85% of predicted, these patients still had abnormalities in expiratory flow rates with and FEV_1/FVC equal to 0.64. At this point, despite the persistent obstructive defect, ipratropium produced only a mild, 6% improvement in FEV_1.

Bronchial Hyperresponsiveness

The recent observation of bronchial hyperresponsiveness (BHR) in patients with heart failure provides evidence that the baseline state of the airways is abnormal making them more reactive to various stimuli.[50–54] It should be noted that not all studies have shown this,[55,56] but the majority of clinical studies have demonstrated some degree of BHR in patients with decompensated as well as compensated CHF. The pathophysiology underlying BHR in these patients remains open to debate. Possible mechanisms are presented below.

Increased Bronchial Smooth Muscle Tone. Vagal contribution to BHR has been suggested by the finding in dogs that histamine enhances reductions in dynamic compliance and increases in airway resistance associated with acute pulmonary vascular congestion—an effect that can be blocked by vagotomy.[57] Brunnee and colleagues[52] found complete reversibility of the increased responsiveness to acetylcholine with the β-agonist, salbutamol, suggesting that the BHR was secondary to an increase in bronchial smooth muscle tone. Of note, they also saw a tendency for BHR in patients treated with an angiotensin-converting enzyme (ACE) inhibitor making a role for the kinin system a possibility.

Bronchial Vascular Congestion and Bronchial Wall Swelling. An additional mechanism is implied from work by Cabanes et al.[50] in which they showed significant BHR to methacholine in a series of patients with New York Heart Association (NYHA) class III heart failure. Consistent with the study by Brunnee[52] they found reversibility with a β-agonist, however in this case, it was only partial. The novel finding was that pretreatment with methoxamine, and α-adrenergic agonist and therefore, a vasoconstrictor as well as a mild bronchoconstrictor, completely prevented the effects of methacholine. These findings suggest then that bronchial vascular congestion with consequent bronchial wall swelling plays a role in BHR either directly[58] or indirectly by stimulation of vagal afferents or by effects on smooth muscle tone. In any event, methoxamine would exert a beneficial effect by reduction of vascular engorgement.[50] An interesting sidelight is that the inhalation of methoxamine prior to exercise in CHF enhanced performance implying that exercise-induced vasodilatation within the bronchial walls contributes to exertional dyspnea.[51]

This last mechanism suggested for BHR may also explain the observation that vasodilators may produce a paradoxical increase in peripheral airways resistance despite a fall in pulmonary vascular pressure. Such a phenomenon is illustrated in Figure 2. One might expect that methoxamine

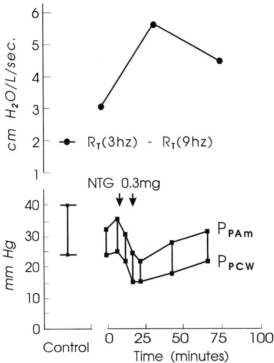

Figure 2. Response to sublingual nitroglycerin (NTG) in a 59-year-old man with an acute myocardial infarction (AMI). Frequency dependence of total respiratory airflow resistance, measured by the oscillometric technique and expressed as the difference between the value at 3hz and 9 hz, R_T(3 hz) - R_T(9 hz), is plotted along with mean pulmonary artery pressure (P_{PAm}) and wedge pressure (P_{PCW}). This frequency dependence of R_T, thought to reflect small airway resistance, is directly correlated with pulmonary vascular pressure under steady state conditions in patients with AMI,[8] but with acute vasodilatation there was a paradoxical increase in frequency dependence of R_T as pulmonary vascular pressure decreased. This could reflect either compression of small airways in the bronchovascular compartment due to dilatation of pulmonary arterioles or bronchial mucosal congestion due to vasodilatation in the bronchial circulation.

could have similar beneficial effects in this clinical situation as described in Cabanes's series of patients.

Respiratory Muscle Function in CHF

The importance of respiratory muscle strength is becoming increasingly recognized in a wide range of respiratory disorders. Numerous studies have shown respiratory muscle weakness in patients with heart failure.[59-64] Hammond et al.[59] compared maximal inspiratory pressure (Pi_{max}), maximal expiratory pressure (Pe_{max}), and maximal handgrip force in patients with heart failure to age matched control subjects. They found significant reductions in both Pi_{max} and Pe_{max} and less dramatic but significant reductions in hand grip strength. The authors pointed out that the respiratory muscle weakness appeared out of proportion to the hand grip weakness and proposed compromised blood flow to the respiratory muscles as the probable mechanism. Other studies have also documented reductions in Pi_{max} and Pe_{max} and correlated them with the severity of functional status.[60] In addition, Pi_{max} has been positively correlated with cardiac index and maximal oxygen consumption making inspiratory muscle weakness a likely contributor to the limitation of exercise in patients with chronic CHF.[61]

Mancini and coworkers[64] used near-infrared spectroscopy to measure oxygenation of the serratus anterior muscle during exercise.[64] With increasing workload they found evidence of muscle deoxygenation in patients with CHF, but not control subjects, suggesting hypoperfusion of accessory muscles of respiration with stress. These same investigators[62] studied diaphragmatic function in patients with moderate heart failure during exercise. They found that although diaphragmatic fatigue does not occur, diaphragmatic work was significantly greater than controls at rest and at all levels of exercise approaching levels of work known to produce fatigue. In addition, they observed significant correlations between respiratory muscle function and the patients' sense of dyspnea.

Acute decompensation resulting in increased work of breathing may magnify latent respiratory muscle weakness potentially leading to hypercapnic respiratory failure. In a canine model of cardiogenic shock it has been demonstrated that respiratory muscle fatigue and respiratory failure is the immediate cause of death.[65] After the reduction in cardiac output there is an initial increase in the strength of diaphragmatic contraction. This is followed by a progressive decrease in the tension developed during inspiration despite increased electrical activity in the electromyograph (EMG) and phrenic neurogram. If the animal is ventilated, death due to cardiogenic shock is avoided and the development of lactic acidosis is much less severe.[66]

Pulmonary Vascular Changes

An understanding of the pathophysiologic changes that occur in the pulmonary vascular system provides further insight into many of the clinical and radiographic findings in patients with CHF.

Pulmonary Vascular Compliance and Volume

In CHF there is an increase in P_{LA} that is reflected passively in a retrograde fashion to the pulmonary veins, capillaries, and arteries. This results in an increase in pulmonary vascular distending pressure with consequent effects on pulmonary blood volume (PBV) that depend on the compliance of the pulmonary vasculature. Intuitively, an increase in distending pressure would be expected to cause an increase in PBV, but the findings of Schreiner et al.[67] indicate that this is not always the case. They demonstrated that the change in vascular volume is dependent on the severity of CHF as assessed by the NYHA functional class. In patients with NYHA class I and II CHF, they found little change in PBV, whereas in NYHA class III patients there was left atrial hypertension and an increase in PBV presumably due to the recruitment of closed vascular units or distension of existing ones. In contrast, patients with NYHA class IV, the distending effects of left atrial hypertension on PBV were outweighed by restriction of the pulmonary vascular bed leading to a reduction in PBV. This implies that pulmonary vascular compliance is influenced by the duration and severity of elevations in vascular pressures. These hemodynamic findings are consistent with the morphologic observation that pathologic changes of intimal fibrosis and medial hypertrophy occur when pulmonary arteries and veins are exposed to increased intraluminal pressures over time.[68]

Pulmonary Blood Flow Distribution

Elevation of pulmonary venous pressure is accompanied by a fairly characteristic redistribution of pulmonary blood flow. This redistribution is such that the lung bases, which normally receive the highest blood flow, experience a decrease in blood flow while the apices, which normally receive the least amount of flow, experience an increase in blood flow. The earliest descriptions of gravitational flow redistribution in patients with elevated pulmonary venous pressure came from studies of patients with mitral stenosis using radionuclide imaging.[69,70] Friedman and Braunwald[70] showed that the ratio of radioactivity between the upper and lower thirds (U/L ratio) of the lung in the erect position was approximately 2:5 in normal subjects compared to 1:1 in patients with mitral stenosis. The U/L ratio was also closely correlated with mean P_{LA}. This flow redistribution, which can be demonstrated by radionuclide imaging, is the basis for the radiographic changes in CHF known as "cephalization," which include engorged upper lobe vessels and narrowed ill-defined lower lobe vessels.[71–73]

The mechanism underlying redistribution involves relative changes in pulmonary vascular resistance (PVR) within the various lung regions. Insight was initially provided by West et al.[74] using an isolated dog lung preparation. They found that raising venous pressures caused increased PVR in the dependent zone of the isolated lung that was felt to be secondary to perivascular interstitial edema. They postulated that the site of increased PVR was in the extra-alveolar vessels where interstitial edema blunted the tethering action that the lung parenchyma exerts on these microvessels to keep them open. In accordance with this, increasing lung volumes and transpulmonary pressures, which cause a reduction in interstitial pressure and extra-alveolar vessel resistance, reverse the degree of basal to apical flow redistribution both in the isolated dog lung[75] and in healthy human subjects.[76]

From these studies came the paradigm that the flow to the most dependent lung zones is determined by the arterial-interstitial pressure gradient (so-called zone 4) rather than the arterial-venous pressure gradient or arterial-alveolar pressure gradient, which determines flow to zones 1, 2, and 3 of West.[77] When interstitial pressure is elevated by edema and increased vascular pressure, flow to an increased proportion of the lung is governed by this zone 4 phenomenon producing the characteristic changes in blood flow distribution seen in patients with CHF.

Hughes et al.[78] evaluated regional pulmonary blood flow in the upright position in both patients with elevated P_{LA} and in normal subjects. In both groups of subjects there were regions of reduced blood flow at the base of the lung and the level of maximum regional flow moved toward the apex at lower lung volumes. In patients with elevated P_{LA} the level at which maximal blood flow occurred at both FRC and TLC was 6 cm more cephalad than in the normal subjects. This cephalad displacement of the level for maximal blood flow indicates a greater amount of the lung being perfused under zone 4 conditions in the patients with increased P_{LA}. Of significance, the extent of zone 4 appeared to correlate with P_{LA} and, by inference to interstitial pressure, adding credence to the notion that an increase in interstitial pressure is a critical factor in the determination of zone 4 and blood flow redistribution.

Other factors that influence regional blood in flow CPE include atelectasis, alveolar hypoxia, and alveolar edema.[79–81] All of these would be expected to redistribute flow away from affected areas. Such effects are not unique to CPE since there are studies in low pressure edema that indicate blood flow redistribution away from the most severely injured and edematous regions.[82–84]

Modulation of the defect in gas exchange that accompanies CHF is one area in which pulmonary blood flow redistribution becomes particularly important. Perfusion of the pulmonary capillaries in edema filled or collapsed alveoli has the effect of a right to left shunt because venous blood that is not exposed to alveolar air is admixed with oxygenated blood from ventilated alveoli. If 50% of the alveoli are filled with edema fluid and these alveoli were perfused at the same rate as functioning alveoli, the arterial PO_2 would be severely reduced just as it would be in the presence of a 50% shunt. Conversely, perfusion redistribution limiting flow to the edematous alveoli to 30% of cardiac output (CO) would minimize the severity of arterial hypoxemia, making it equivalent to a 30% shunt. As will be discussed later, vasodilator therapy for CHF while improving cardiac function may increase the severity of hypoxemia by reversing pulmonary blood flow redistribution.[85–87] Alkalosis by attenuation of hypoxic pulmonary vasoconstriction can have a similar effect on flow redistribution and gas exchange.[88–91]

Radiographic Manifestations of CHF

The radiographic manifestations are determined by the stage in the evolution of pulmonary edema that predominates at a given time. For instance, the radiograph of a patient with primarily interstitial edema has different characteristics than one in which alveolar edema or pulmonary congestion is the major abnormality. Common to all of these stages, however, is blood flow redistribution from basal to apical regions producing the characteristic cephalization of the pulmonary vasculature.[71] In mitral stenosis there is good correlation between the severity of radiographic findings and vascular pressures.[70] Such a relationship, has also been suggested for patients with myocardial infarction.[92] When the radiographic data are examined in terms of their predictive power, however, the picture is less clear. Chakko et al.[93] studied patients with chronic CHF referred for evaluation for heart transplantation and reported that conventional clinical and radiographic signs of heart failure had a poor predictive value for identifying patients with elevated pulmonary capillary wedge pressure (P_{PCW}). They found that 53% of patients with P_{PCW} between 16 and 29 mm Hg and 39% of patients with P_{PCW} >30 mm Hg did not have radiographic findings of pulmonary congestion. A similar lack of predictive value for the radiographic findings in AMI is illustrated in Figure 3.

The discordance between vascular pressures, the degree of alveolar edema and radiographic findings has supported the concept of temporal phase lags.[92,94,95] The fact that mitral stenosis is marked by chronic elevation of P_{LA} producing a relatively static situation may explain why there is a better correlation in radiographic and hemodynamic parameters; whereas, a condition characterized by rapid changes in vascular pressures such as in myocardial infarction is more prone to phase lags. As a result of phase lags, one may see a patient with markedly elevated P_{LA} but potentially very little evidence of interstitial or alveolar edema depending on the duration of the elevated P_{LA}, hence, the apparent discrepancy in the patient's clinical status

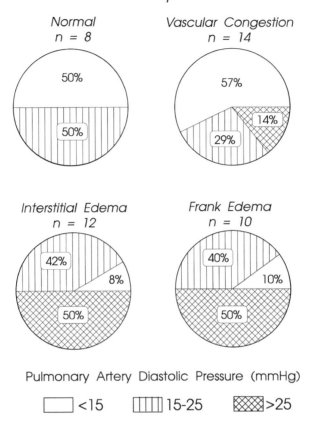

Pulmonary Artery Diastolic Pressure (mmHg)

☐ <15   ⊞ 15-25   ▓ >25

Figure 3. Relationship between radiologic findings and pulmonary hemodynamics in 44 patients with acute myocardial infarction. Portable chest radiographs read by staff radiologists, without knowledge of hemodynamic measurements, are compared to the pulmonary diastolic (P_{PAd}) pressures measured at the time of the radiologic examination. Positive predictive value (PPV) is the probability of a certain hemodynamic finding based on the radiologic diagnosis (true positives/total positives). Negative predictive value (NPV) is the probability of excluding a certain hemodynamic finding based on the radiologic diagnosis (true negatives/total negatives).

RADIOLOGIC DIAGNOSIS	P_{PAd}	>15 mm Hg	P_{PAd}	>25 mmHg
Predictive Value	PPV	NPV	PPV	NPV
Pulmonary Vascular Congestion	43%	50%	14%	100%
Interstitial Pulmonary Edema	92%	55%	50%	91%
Frank Pulmonary Edema	90%	38%	50%	76%

For example, if the radiograph shows interstitial edema this indicates P_{PAd} >15 with 92% certainty or P_{PAd} >25 with 50% certainty. Conversely, if the radiograph shows no interstitial edema, i.e. it is normal or shows only vascular congestion this excludes P_{PAd} >15 with 55% certainty or P_{PAd} >25 with 91% certainty. Clearly a radiographic diagnosis of "Pulmonary Vascular Congestion" is of little help except in the exclusion of P_{PAd} >25, and the diagnosis of either "Interstitial Edema" or "Frank Pulmonary Edema" is useful only in that it indicates P_{PAd} >15 with reasonable certainty. The distinction between "Interstitial Edema" and "Frank Pulmonary Edema" was of no value in the estimation of P_{PAd}. (Data are from Biddle et al.[235]).

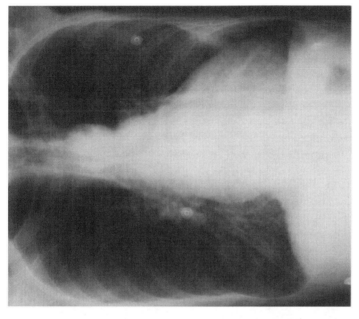

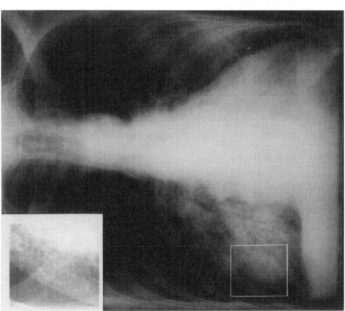

Figure 4. Chest radiographs taken at this time of hospital admission (left) and two days later (right) in a patient with a history of both CHF and chronic obstructive pulmonary disease. The admission diagnosis was bacterial pneumonia. The film on the right shows almost miraculous clearing of the pneumonic infiltrate after 2 days of antibiotic therapy. In addition to antibiotics the treatment had included bed rest, oxygen, and furosemide, at 80 mg per day. In retrospect, close inspection of the admission radiograph reveals Kerley B lines (see inset).

and their radiograph. Conversely, after treatment, P_{LA} may be reduced, but radiographic improvement may be significantly delayed.[94]

Another source for the discrepancy between radiographic and hemodynamic findings is the variability in the relationship between lung water accumulation and pulmonary vascular pressure. Using positron emission tomographic imaging methods in patients with CHF it has been shown that variability of P_{PCW} between patients can account for only 22% of the variability in lung water.[96] Clearly a part of this variability relates to the duration of P_{LA} elevation, the temporal phase lag concept. Other sources of variability are related to the factors that determine the relationship between lung water balance and microvascular pressure. These are discussed in Chapter 2. Even in a given patient there may be regional variability in the relationship between edema and vascular pressure leading to segmental or lobar infiltrates that may be misdiagnosed as pneumonia.[97] Chest radiographs to illustrate this point are shown in Figure 4. This patient, with a history of both CHF and chronic obstructive pulmonary disease, was misdiagnosed with pneumonia and experienced a dramatic response to antibiotic therapy. Of course the treatment also included bed rest, oxygen, and furosemide at 80 mg per day. It appears that prior lung disease may have altered the relationship between vascular pressure and regional lung water accumulation either through changes in capillary surface area or lymphatic function.

Gas Exchange

Arterial hypoxemia is the major gas exchange abnormality that develops in nearly all patients with CHF and the severity of hypoxemia is closely related to the severity of LV failure. Acid-base abnormalities in patients with CHF range from mild respiratory alkalosis to severe respiratory acidosis often combined with metabolic acidosis.

Hypoxemia

The principle mechanism of hypoxemia in patients with CHF depends on the stage of pulmonary edema. In mild CHF with only interstitial edema airway closure leads to ventilation/perfusion (V/Q) mismatch and hypoxemia on that basis. In severe CHF with alveolar edema, intrapulmonary shunt is the major mechanism of hypoxemia. Changes in cardiac output can modify the severity of hypoxemia both through a direct effect on mixed venous O_2 content and through an indirect effect on perfusion distribution. Except in severe cases, diffusion impairment rarely contributes to hypoxemia.

Airway Closure and V/Q Mismatch

The etiology for hypoxemia in interstitial edema relates to premature airway closure and ventilation-perfusion mismatch. Premature airway closure as evidenced by elevated closing volume has been discussed above in the setting of myocardial infarction and volume loading. A clear understanding of what closing volume is in physiologic terms is essential to appreciating how elevated CV can affect gas exchange in heart failure. It is important to distinguish between residual volume and CV. While in young healthy subjects residual volume is determined by the minimum configuration of the chest wall, in older subjects residual volume is determined by expiratory flow limitation and airway closure.[98] Under these conditions, residual volume is the lung volume at which all airways are, in effect, closed. During exhalation, residual volume is approached, airway closure occurs in lower lung regions and CV is the lung volume, above residual volume, at which airway closure begins. Elevated CV develops when interstitial pressure is increased by loss of elastic recoil or interstitial edema or when there is small airway dysfunction. Airway closure occurs in dependent lung zones, where transpulmonary distending pressure is lowest and interstitial pressure is greatest resulting in a shift of ventilation from these dependent areas to upper lung zones.

The effect of premature airway closure on gas exchange depends on the relationship between closing volume and the end-expiratory lung volume, FRC. In healthy people, closing volume is less than expiratory reserve volume (RV) and the absolute lung volume at which airway closure occurs, called closing capacity (CC),

$$CC = RV + CV \tag{1}$$

remains, for the most part, below FRC and therefore does not have functional significance during tidal breathing. In patients with CC elevated above FRC, the portion of each tidal breath inspired at lung volumes below CC is delivered only to those upper regions with open airways and in the lower lung zones with closed airways there is no inspired ventilation until lung volume exceeds CC. The perfusion of these regions results in lung units with low (but finite) V/Q ratios and hypoxemia. It follows that hypoxemia should correlate with the degree that CC is elevated above FRC.[99] Such a relationship was noted by Jones et al.[100] in a study of dogs with experimental pulmonary vascular congestion in which they observed a correlation between the difference between CC and FRC and the alveolar-arterial PO_2 gradient ($AaDO_2$). As this difference increased, the $AaDO_2$ widened. This rationale also applies to the hypoxemia seen when subjects are given a rapid infusion of saline or in the setting of AMI because a fall in

FRC often occurs in these situations.[10–12] It should be noted that there does not have to be an increase in CC for there to be significant hypoxemia as a result of airway closure at lung volumes above FRC. In fact there is a significant correlation between PaO_2 and the reduction in FRC after AMI in the absence of any detectable change in closing volume.[10,17]

Intrapulmonary Shunt

Whereas alveolar edema is an obvious cause of intrapulmonary shunt in patients with more severe degrees of CHF, atelectasis should not be overlooked. Reduced surfactant activity, which can be demonstrated in experimental animals with pulmonary edema[101] is probably the major cause of atelectasis in patients with CPE, but absorption atelectasis in low V/Q alveoli during O_2 supplementation[102] probably also occurs. These types of atelectatsis are readily reversible and their importance in any given patient can be demonstrated by observing the change in oxygenation that occurs with several minutes of deep breathing. If this is done after the patient has been breathing $100\%O_2$ for 10–20 minutes, so that shunting is the only possible cause for hypoxemia, the increase in PaO_2 is considerable with changes as great as 100 mm Hg. If the shunt is measured, the decrease in Qs/Qt produced by this maneuver may be as large as 10%–20% of the cardiac output.[103–105] In patients who are unable to increase their tidal volume spontaneously, a similar increase in oxygenation can be accomplished through increased tidal volume produced by treatment with intermittent positive pressure breathing.[106] Intubation and mechanical ventilation with positive end-expiratory pressure (PEEP), or continuous positive airway pressure (CPAP) breathing by face mask,[107–110] can have a similar effect through the reversal of atelectasis, but PEEP and CPAP may have additional beneficial influences on oxygenation through the redistribution of edema fluid out of the alveolar space and into the peribronchial interstitial space.[111] The beneficial effects of positive airway pressure are not limited to an improvement in gas exchange. There can be additional benefits derived from changes in the work of breathing and LV mechanics (*vide infra*).

Diffusing Capacity

The effect of CHF on the diffusing capacity appears to be minimal as most studies have not reported significant alterations.[18,46] The competing factors of pulmonary venous congestion with an increased pulmonary capillary blood volume that would increase diffusion capacity lung carbon monoxide (D_LCO), and interstitial/alveolar edema that would decrease

D_LCO, may serve to negate one another.[112] Thus, as in most other disorders of the lung, it is unlikely that diffusion limitation contributes to hypoxemia at rest in patients with CHF. The balance between these factors in a given patient may however vary depending on their clinical state with decompensated patients in pulmonary edema tending to have lower diffusing capacities. This is shown by Siegel et al.[113] who found that D_LCO/VA is significantly reduced in patients with rales compared to those without rales despite having similar ejection fractions. This led them to conclude that D_LCO is a good predictor of clinically evident heart failure. In general, though, in the absence of frank pulmonary edema a low D_LCO should alert the clinician to the possibility of underlying lung or pulmonary vascular disease. In patients with mitral stenosis a fall in diffusing capacity usually indicates the onset of reactive pulmonary hypertension.[114,115]

Influence of Cardiac Output

Another major cause of hypoxemia that should not be overlooked is a reduced cardiac output. Its potential impact on gas exchange is demonstrated by the relationship of arterial PO_2 to the spectrum of hemodynamic changes that can occur with myocardial infarction ranging from uncomplicated to CHF (Killip class I) to cardiogenic shock (class IV). Most studies[116–119] have shown that the most severe arterial hypoxemia occurs in cardiogenic shock compared to the other clinical states. Mackenzie et al.[116] reported an average PaO_2 of 47 mmHg for those in shock with some patients presenting with values <40 mmHg. Characteristically, this profound hypoxemia is less responsive to increasing F_1O_2 compared to that observed in patients without shock.[116–119] These observations highlight the point that the effect of an intrapulmonary shunt is enhanced in a low cardiac output state. While reduced cardiac output should not increase the shunt, it will increase the effect on PaO_2. On the other hand there is evidence that increases in CO can increase the fraction of CO traversing the intrapulmonary shunt, through blood flow redistribution. Thus, the overall influence of changes in cardiac output on arterial oxygenation depend on the balance between changes in percent of flow shunted and the direct influence of the shunt on PaO_2.

The influence of cardiac output on the severity of arterial hypoxemia in the presence of a shunt follows directly from the Fick equation:

$$O_2 \text{ consumption } (\dot{V}O_2) = CO(CaO_2\text{-}CvO_2) \tag{2}$$

To maintain a particular $\dot{V}O_2$ in the setting of reduced CO the arterial-mixed venous O_2 content difference (CaO_2-CvO_2) must widen and this can only occur with a reduction in CvO_2. In the presence of a shunt, arterial blood is a mixture of well oxygenated blood from the capillaries of ventilated alveoli and mixed venous blood. Consequently CaO_2, and therefore PaO_2, are determined both by the size of the shunt and by the CvO_2. This effect is illustrated in Figure 5. The influence of CO on PaO_2 in the presence of a given shunt is an important principle for the development of therapeutic strategies. Figure 6 illustrates this relationship at two different F_IO_2. The key point is that the importance of cardiac output for arterial oxygenation increases as the size of the shunt increases. This is true whether F_IO_2 is 21% or 100% but the response to O_2 is greater the greater the CO.

As mentioned above this direct effect of cardiac output on PaO_2 can be modulated by changes in the size of the intrapulmonary shunt. A number of studies indicate that reduced cardiac output can decrease the fraction of pulmonary blood flow traversing the shunt.[106,120–123] Scheinman and Evans[106] observed a mean shunt fraction of 11% in patients with myocardial infarction and clinical evidence of shock contrasted with a mean shunt fraction of 16% in those without shock. Such a relationship has also been shown experimentally by Lynch et al.[120] who manipulated the cardiac output in dogs with oleic acid induced pulmonary edema and examined the subsequent effect on intrapulmonary shunt. They found a consistent and reproducible association between changes in cardiac output and intrapulmonary shunt fraction regardless of whether the cardiac output was manipulated by

Shunt = 20%

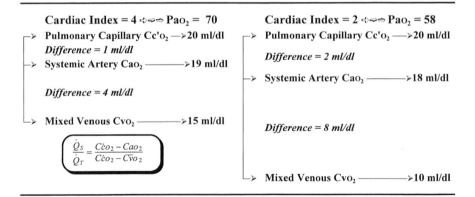

Figure 5. The determinants of CaO_2 and PaO_2 when breathing air with a 20% shunt. Notice that the difference between pulmonary capillary and arterial blood is 20% of the difference between pulmonary capillary and mixed venous O_2 contents. When the cardiac index is reduced from 4 to 2 L/min/m² the arterial - venous O_2 difference increases from 4 to 8 mL/dL (VO_2=160 mL/min/m²), and the decrease in CvO_2 leads to corresponding reductions in CaO_2 and PaO_2. The ($Cc'O_2$ - CaO_2) difference is directly proportional to (CaO_2 - CvO_2).

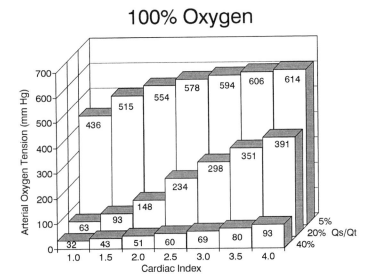

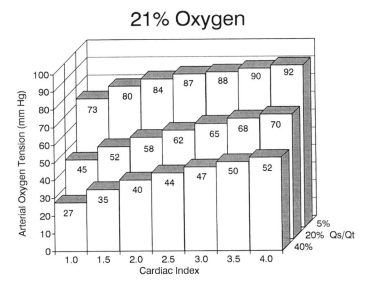

Figure 6. The relationship between shunt (Qs/Qt), cardiac index (CI), F_IO_2 and arterial PO_2. Notice that the PaO_2 is relatively insensitive to changes in CI when Qs/Qt is normal (5%), but with increase in Qs/Qt, changes in the CI have more influence on PaO_2. For example PaO_2 is only 40 when shunt is 40% and CI is 2 and the patient is breathing air. If the F_IO_2 is increased to 100% the PaO_2 would increase to 51. This may be an important increase in oxygenation, but therapy to decrease the shunt to 20% would increase the PaO_2 to 148 on 100% O_2, or therapy to increase the CI to 3.0 would increase the PaO_2 to 69 on 100% O_2.

mechanical or pharmacologic means. The same relationship between CO and CvO_2, may explain the changes in intrapulmonary shunt with changes in CO. While some[106] have postulated that channels through edematous and atelectatic lung tissue possess a higher vascular resistance and are therefore progressively recruited at higher cardiac outputs, Dantzker[122] has advanced the theory that the changes are related to modulation of hypoxic pulmonary vasoconstriction by the PO_2 of mixed venous blood. Reductions in PvO_2 increase vascular resistance of these channels whereas increases in PvO_2 decrease their resistance leading to changes in fractional shunt, which parallels changes in CO. Whether modulation of hypoxic vasoconstriction is the whole explanation has been questioned by other studies.[124–126]

Relationship to Pulmonary Hemodynamics

Given the mechanics reviewed above, it is not surprising that several studies have demonstrated a significant relationship between arterial hypoxemia and pulmonary vascular pressure elevation. This has been particularly notable in patients with AMI.[8,10,105,127–129] Figure 7 illustrates this cor-

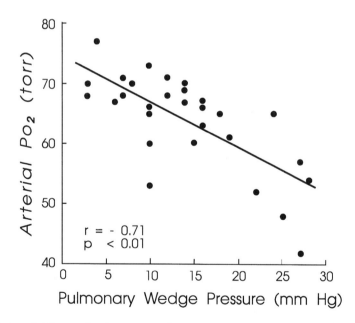

Figure 7. Arterial PO_2 and pulmonary wedge pressure measurements in 29 patients with acute myocardial infarction. The measurements were obtained breathing air. The negative correlation between PaO_2 and P_{PCW} is shown. (Data are from Interiano et al.[8] and Gray et al.[10])

relation in a group of patients with acute myocardial infarction. A similar relationship has been observed in normal subjects given acute volume expansion with dextran.[12] In these studies, the rapid infusion of dextran sufficient to increase P_{PCW} 11 mmHg resulted in a reduction in PaO_2 of 14 mmHg. Finally, in mitral stenosis, Friedman et al.[130] found that hypoxemia correlated with the severity of the valvular disease. Clearly when the elevation in P_{LA} is sufficient to produce alveolar flooding this could be the mechanism for the correlation. With smaller increases in P_{LA} it has been suggested that the mechanism is the reduction in FRC leading to airway closure at lung volumes within the tidal range.[10,17] The relationship between $AaDO_2$ and FRC following acute myocardial infarction (AMI) and after recovery is shown in Figure 8.

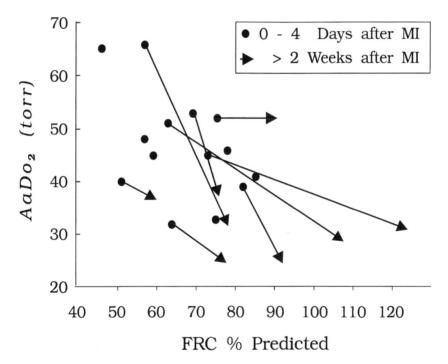

Figure 8. The alveolar - arterial PO_2 difference ($AaDO_2$) is plotted against FRC for 14 patients during the first four days after acute myocardial infarction. Follow up measurements were made in eight patients after hospital discharge. All measurements were made in the semi-recumbent posture with the patient breathing air. Circles indicate the acute period and triangles indicate studies after recovery. With recovery from AMI all patients experienced an increase in FRC and all but one experienced a decrease in the $AaDO_2$. (Data are from Gray et al.[10])

Acid Base Alterations

While respiratory alkalosis is the most common alteration seen in patients with CHF, respiratory acidosis frequently combined with metabolic acidosis is the most challenging management problem.[131,132] The distribution of acid-base disturbances in heart failure was described by O'Donovan et al.[133] in 81 patients presenting with cardiogenic pulmonary edema. The results were as follows: 23% had no acid-base disturbance; 41%, isolated respiratory alkalosis; 22%, metabolic acidosis; 10%, metabolic alkalosis; 9%, respiratory acidosis. Surprisingly, in this series of patients, acid-base abnormalities did not predict mortality, morbidity, or the severity of the pulmonary edema.

Respiratory and Metabolic Acidosis

An earlier retrospective study described a somewhat higher percentage of patients, 50% presenting with respiratory acidosis frequently complicated by coexisting metabolic acidosis.[131] These data were collected in 1967, an era before blood gas analysis became routine, and may reflect the selection of only the sicker patients for this procedure. However, in a prospective study Aberman and Fullop,[132] found that 43 of 46 patients with acute cardiogenic pulmonary edema had metabolic acidosis. While only 25% of the patients had elevated PCO_2, many of those with normal PCO_2 had uncompensated metabolic acidosis, which also indicates relative alveolar hypoventilation. They also found that respiratory acidosis did not predict a poor outcome even when the treatment included morphine and high flow oxygen, interventions usually avoided in the treatment of patients with hypercapnia from other causes. In fact, the patients generally responded rapidly to conventional therapy with only one of eleven hypercapnic patients requiring assisted ventilation. Even with these observations of respiratory acidosis as a consequence of heart failure, the clinician should be careful to exclude other forms of lung disease in the hypercapnic patient. If pulmonary edema is the primary etiology the hypercapnia should be acute, with no evidence of renal compensation, and should resolve promptly with effective treatment of the heart failure.

Dead Space Ventilation. Increased physiologic dead space may also play a role in the relative alveolar hypoventilation seen in some patients with pulmonary edema. Besides increased $AaDO_2$, increased physiologic dead space (Vd/Vt) is another manifestation of V/Q inhomogeneity. Early in the evolution of heart failure, there may be an improvement in the V/Q matching and a reduction in Vd/Vt owing to redistribution of blood flow to the well ventilated but relatively underperfused upper lung zones. In clinical practice, though, other factors usually intervene and Vd/Vt may be unchanged or increased in heart failure. Saunders[134] found an increased Vd/Vt in only 8 of 26 patients with left ventricular failure (LVF) after taking into account changes in respiratory rate and tidal volume. Notably, with clinical recovery, he reported that Vd/Vt either increased or remained unchanged. This observation prompted Saunders[134] to conclude that LVF per se does not produce an increase in Vd/Vt. The reported changes in physiologic dead space in the setting of myocardial infarction conflict somewhat with those expected from Saunders's conclusions. Numerous studies in patients with AMI have reported an increased Vd/Vt.[104,128,135,136] Data from Higgs[104] indicate that these changes are most evident in the presence of pulmonary congestion. Furthermore, Tattersfield et al.[128] found that there was a direct correlation between pulmonary artery pressure (P_{PA}) and Vd/Vt, but the Vd/Vt was only modestly elevated, 0.39, in this group of patients with AMI and reasonably normal tidal volume, 600 mL. The possibility that the increase in Vd/Vt in patients with elevated vascular pressures or pulmonary congestion could be partially explained by more rapid respiration in those with worse LVF should, however, be kept in mind.

A rise in Vd/Vt in response to exercise in patients with chronic heart failure is well documented and is considered an important contributing factor to their exercise limitation.[137–141] Exercise testing in these patients has revealed an inverse relationship between the Vd/Vt and cardiac output.[138] Accordingly, it has been advocated that the pattern of ventilatory changes with exercise testing provides an accurate and objective assessment of CHF severity.[139] In addition to a reduced cardiac output with exercise, other proposed mechanisms for the increased Vd/Vt include chronic pulmonary vasculature changes secondary to chronic congestion and the development of rapid shallow breathing secondary to stimulation of mechanoreceptors and reduced lung compliance.

Respiratory Alkalosis

Whereas the hypercapnia of respiratory acidosis will decrease arterial PO_2 by decreasing alveolar PO_2, respiratory alkalosis should improve PaO_2 by an opposite effect on alveolar PO_2. However, instead of improving, oxygenation alkalosis may contribute to tissue hypoxia through two mechanisms. First, alkalosis has been associated with an increase in V/Q mismatch and intrapulmonary shunt. Second, alkalosis has several different effects on the oxygen-hemoglobin dissociation curve, which determine the availability of O_2 for any given PaO_2.

Although the effect of alkalosis on V/Q mismatch and intrapulmonary shunt is most often described for metabolic alkalosis,[142] this phenomenon has also been noted with respiratory alkalosis.[143] The mechanism involves attenuation of hypoxic pulmonary vasoconstriction, which leads to increased perfusion of poorly or unventilated alveoli.[88–91] The potential clinical relevance of these changes was illustrated by Brimioulle et al.[144] who found worsening V/Q matching with metabolic alkalosis in patients with shunt fraction >20% and significant improvement in PaO_2 from 65 to 100 mmHg after correction with hydrochloric acid (HCl) administration.

Tissue Oxygenation

Tissue oxygenation depends on the oxygen content of arterial blood, cardiac output, and oxyhemoglobin dissociation at the tissue level. This latter issue has been examined in both acute myocardial infarction[145] and chronic cardiac failure.[146] With reduced cardiac output oxygen consumption is maintained by increased oxygen extraction, which is facilitated by an adaptive decrease in oxygen - hemoglobin affinity. Oxygen - hemoglobin affinity is quantified as P_{50}, the PO_2 at 50% saturation. An increase in P_{50} signifies a decrease in affinity or a shift of the dissociation curve to the right, which will increase venous PO_2, and tissue PO_2.

With changes in acid base balance it is important to distinguish between P_{50} std and P_{50} in vivo. P_{50} std indicates the position of the dissociation curve corrected to pH 7.4, PCO_2 40, and temperature 37°C. P_{50} in vivo is the position of the curve at the pH, PCO_2, and temperature existing in the patient. An increase in P_{50} std is caused by an increase in red cell 2,3-diphosphoglycerate (2,3-DPG). Although an increase in 2,3-DPG usually accompanies reductions in tissue oxygenation caused by anemia, altitude, or low cardiac output,[147] alkalosis is also usually present under these conditions. In the absence of alkalosis there is little increase in 2,3-DPG and alkalosis, by itself, can cause an increase in P_{50} std over the period of 24–48 hours.[148] This effect is directly opposite to the reduction in P_{50} in vivo produced by acute alkalosis through the Bohr effect. Thus with prolonged alkalosis the Bohr effect and the slowly developing increase in 2,3-DPG tend to offset each other. Despite these confounding factors it is possible to demonstrate that P_{50} increases in proportion to the severity of cardiac failure in patients with AMI. In uncomplicated AMI (Killip class I) P_{50} std and P_{50} in vivo are 26.9 and 26.0 torr, respectively (normal = 26.8). In the presence of pulmonary edema (class III) the same values are increased to 31.2 and 31.4 torr. Intermediate values of 28.7 and 28.0 are found in mild CHF (class II) without pulmonary edema. This progression did not extend to patients with cardiogenic shock (class IV) where both values were in the normal range, 26.8 and 27.1, possibly as the result of less alkalosis. Similar decreases in oxygen - hemoglobin affinity to facilitate tissue oxygenation are found in chronic CHF.[146]

Treatment

Because of the interdependence of the cardiovascular and respiratory systems, therapy directed at one system can potentially have beneficial or adverse effects on the other system, which may serve to limit its application depending on the physiologic status of the patient. In the preceding sections we have made reference to the response to therapy when this clarifies a physiologic mechanism. In this section, we will review various conventional as well as newer modalities of therapy for CHF with an emphasis on cardiorespiratory interaction. A comprehensive review of all of the newer modalities of hemodynamic therapy with no known or expected effect on the respiratory system is beyond the scope of this chapter.

Oxygen

Hypoxemia is an almost constant feature of the pathophysiology of CHF, and pulmonary edema and oxygen supplementation should be the first step in routine management. Of course the response to O_2 therapy will depend on the principle mechanism of hypoxemia and blood gases should be checked to assure that the level of therapy is sufficient. If shunt and/or low cardiac output are the principle mechanisms it will be important to use specific approaches to address these physiologic problems.

Pharmacologic Therapies

Morphine

The beneficial effects of morphine in the treatment of CHF and pulmonary edema have been known for many years. Although morphine sulfate is the mainstay for the treatment of cardiogenic pulmonary edema there is no agreement on the exact physiologic mechanism. The mechanisms proposed include: a) venous pooling due to dilatation of the capacitance vessels; b) reduced left ventricular afterload due to arterial dilatation; and c) respiratory depression leading both to c_1) a decrease in the metabolic load associated with the exaggerated work of breathing and to c_2) a decrease in exaggerated pumping action of the diaphragm, which is thought to facilitate venous return. The hemodynamic effects of morphine could be produced by direct actions on vascular smooth muscle or through modulation of neurogenic vasomotor tone. Although it can be shown that morphine produces reductions in systemic venous tone[149] and splanchnic vasodilatation[150] it has no direct effect on arterial or venous smooth muscle.[151]

Notice that each of the proposed mechanisms involve the cardiovascular system and should reduce LV filling pressure and pulmonary vascular congestion thereby leading to an improvement in respiratory mechanics. It is surprising then that the classic studies of Sharp and coworkers[47] could find no consistent changes in lung compliance or airflow resistance in three patients with moderate pulmonary edema despite subjective improvement following 10 mg of intravenous morphine sulfate. Although the study had certain limitations, the ease with which the physiological benefits from other forms of therapy were detected makes it unlikely that they could have missed a measurable effect of morphine. Even direct measurements of cardiac function in patients with acute myocardial infarction complicated by severe LVF have failed to document improvement in filling pressure after 0.2 mg/kg intravenous morphine sulfate.[152] Some have alluded to the possibility that excessive sympathetic activity may lead to further deterioration of myocardial performance.[153-156] Myocardial oxygen consumption can also be increased from the increased levels of sympathetic tone because of increased heart rate and LV wall tension. Morphine could exert its effect by diminishing this sympathetic activity at a central level, but again one would expect to see an improvement in filling pressures if this is the link between the hemodynamic effects and symptomatic response. Finally, there is the possibility that the sympathetic tone exerts a direct effect on the lung that perpetuates pulmonary edema, i.e. a neurogenic component to cardiogenic pulmonary edema[157] that is blocked by the central sympatholytic action of morphine, but again one would expect to see an improvement in pulmonary mechanics as the edema is ameliorated.

Whatever the mechanism, morphine remains as an important agent for the treatment of acute cardiogenic pulmonary edema and the observations of Aberman and Fulop already discussed[132] make it clear that the existence of hypercapnia is not a contraindication to its use in this setting.

Diuretics

A marked improvement in pulmonary function is usually noted with the use of loop diuretics in the treatment of CHF and pulmonary edema.[135] Furosemide has been noted to illicit a prompt and significant clinical improvement prior to the onset of any significant diuresis.[158] The extrarenal hemodynamic effects of furosemide described by Dikshit and coworkers[159] help to explain the beneficial effects of this diuretic in patients who are in complete anuric renal failure. It is believed to be due to venous vasodilatation, which decreases venous return and left ventricular preload. The loop diuretic ethacrynic acid has a similar immediate effect in the pulmonary circulation[160] where despite reductions in P_{LA} and P_{PA}, pulmonary blood volume is unchanged indicating an increase in pulmonary vascular compliance. While loop diuretics usually increase systemic vascular resistance (SVR) and afterload in euvolemic patients,[161] they have an opposite effect in patients with decompensated CHF and pulmonary edema that may be very prominent and prolonged. It is maximized with a 20 mg dose and is not improved with dosage escalation as opposed to the natriuretic effect that increases in a linear fashion above a threshold dose.[162]

The diuresis produced by the loop diuretics has other effects that are more delayed. The decrease in plasma volume elicited by diuresis causes a decrease in P_{PA} and P_{LA} that should decrease both PBV and EVLW, but these changes are not measurable in the first 60 minutes.[160] In patients with LVF complicating acute myocardial infarction the decrease in EVLW is not detectable until at least 4 hours after the intravenous administration of furosemide.[163] The improvements in gas exchange and reduction in AaDo$_2$ follow a similar time course. While several studies have been unable to demonstrate any consistent improvement in gas exchange for 1–6 hours following the intravenous administration of rapid acting diuretics,[136,164,165] there is one study that demonstrated an improvement at 4 hours, but only in those patients whose initial arterial O$_2$ saturation was below 90%.[135] Measurements obtained 24 hours after diuresis reveal a more consistent improvement in gas exchange.[164] In contrast, improvement in pulmonary mechanics with increases in FEV$_1$ and FVC 4 hours after diuresis was a consistent finding in all patients.[135]

Vasodilators

This class of drugs has proven to be extremely useful in the treatment of CHF and pulmonary edema. In the normal heart, an increase in the SVR results in an increase in the myocardial work and myocardial oxygen consumption with little change in the cardiac output, end-systolic or end-diastolic volumes or pressures. In a diseased heart that is dysfunctional as SVR is increased there are increases in end-systolic and end-diastolic volumes and increased LV end-diastolic pressure and often a decrease in the cardiac output.[166–169]

There are three main subclasses of the vasodilators that are defined by their primary mechanism of action: 1) arterial vasodilators (i.e., hydralazine, alpha 1-receptor antagonists, etc.); 2) venous dilators (i.e., nitroglycerin, isosorbide dinitrate, etc.) and; 3) balanced vasodilators (i.e., ACE inhibitors, nitroprusside, etc.). All three classes of vasodilators are useful in the treatment of myocardial dysfunction. Arterial vasodilators by reducing SVR decrease LV end-systolic and end-diastolic volumes, LVEDP and myocardial wall tension, which is the principal determinant of myocardial oxygen consumption. Venous vasodilators achieve the same end. By reducing filling pressure and end-diastolic volume, they produce secondary reductions in end-systolic volume and myocardial wall tension. For the purpose of this discussion of cardiopulmonary interactions we will focus on the nitrates, which include both venous dilators and balanced vasodilators, and the ACE inhibitors.

Nitrates. Nitroglycerin (NTG) has been used in the treatment of cardiac disease since the mid-19th century. Its original use in cardiac disease was in the treatment of angina pectoris and because of its great success in this condition it rapidly gained widespread acceptance by the medical profession.[170] The list of diseases for which it has been tried is legion. The beneficial effects of NTG on pulmonary vascular pressures in patients with CHF has been known since 1957[171] and it has been shown to be effective for the emergency treatment of cardiogenic pulmonary edema.[172] Sodium nitroprusside (SNP) produces similar changes in pulmonary vascular pressures in this setting,[173,174] but because of a more balanced effect on both the arterial impedance vessels as well as venous capacitance vessels of the systemic circulation SNP also increases cardiac output.[175]

In addition to the actions of the nitrates in the systemic circulation, which produce passive changes in pulmonary vascular pressures, there are also direct effects on the pulmonary circulation, but these effects on the lesser circulation may be difficult to detect because of the larger effects on the greater (systemic) circulation. If blood volume expansion is used to hold P_{PA} and P_{LA} constant during SNP infusion it is possible to demonstrate an increase in PBV and a decrease in PVR in response to SNP.[176] If the responses are studied when vascular tone is increased pharmacologically, both NTG and SNP produce more dramatic decreases in PVR.[177]

These effects of NTG and SNP also operate to reverse hypoxic vasoconstriction in the pulmonary circulation,[178] which can result in increased V/Q mismatch and hypoxemia due to increased perfusion (Q) of regions with low V/Q. This has been demonstrated in animal models of pulmonary edema,[82,87] in healthy human subjects,[179] in patients with CHF,[86] and in other disorders of lung function.[180]

An example of the effects of SNP on cardiac function and gas exchange is provided in Table 1 to provide a sense of the magnitude of the problem. The patient was a 51-year-old white male who had sustained an acute inferior wall myocardial infarction 6 days previously. He had a mild tachycardia, 115, and tachypnea, 27, cold mottled extremities with acrocyanosis, crackles over the lower 2/3 of both lung fields, and a protodiastolic gallop. He was oliguric despite furosemide and had begun to develop azotemia. The chest film revealed diffuse alveolar infiltrates and mild cardiomegaly

_____ **Table 1** _____

Effect of Nitroprusside on Gas Exchange

PaO_2 mmHg	CaO_2-CvO_2 mL/dL	BP mmHg	CI liters/min/m²	P_{PCW} mmHg
	Baseline, O_2 at 2 liters/minute			
105	9.8	110/85	1.6	32
	Nitroprusside 6μg/kg/minute			
51	5.1	115/75	3.1	18

Fifty one year-old-man 6 days after inferior wall myocardial infarction.

consistent with cardiogenic pulmonary edema. Despite the diffuse alveolar edema, gas exchange was good with PaO_2 of 105 mmHg on only 2 L of O_2 by nasal prongs. Right heart catheterization revealed a markedly depressed cardiac index, elevated arterial venous oxygen extraction, and elevated P_{PCW}. Nitroprusside produced a marked clinical improvement without significant change in blood pressure or heart rate. Urine output increased and the extremities became warm. Repeat hemodynamic measurements confirmed the improvement in circulatory status. These data are from a time before the widespread use of pulse oximetry, and if arterial blood gases had not been obtained the significant deterioration in gas exchange would not have been noticed. The PaO_2 had fallen from 105 to 51 mmHg on the same level of O_2 supplementation despite considerable improvement in CvO_2.

The message from this clinical illustration is not to avoid vasodilator therapy, but rather to anticipate deterioration of gas exchange when administering these agents. The F_IO_2 should be increased prophylactically and the PaO_2 closely monitored. If hypoxemia is already a major problem, the potential benefits of vasodilator therapy should be weighed against the risk. Some vasodilators, such as hydralazine,[181] and urapidil, a selective α_1-receptor antagonist,[86] may have less potential for inhibition of hypoxic pulmonary vasoconstriction.

Angiotensin Converting Enzyme Inhibitors. There are no studies that have specifically evaluated the pulmonary consequences of vasodilator therapy with ACE inhibitors. Because of the clear benefit that they have on morbidity and mortality, it is unlikely that there will be any future randomized trials with and without vasodilators to evaluate their effect on pulmonary mechanics and gas exchange.[182–185] It is presumed that the reduction in LV filling pressures and pulmonary vascular pressures would reverse the pathophysiologic processes that promoted the derangements in the pulmonary mechanics and gas exchange. There is direct evidence that ACE inhibitors improve exercise capacity in some patients with myocardial dysfunction and that this effect may be more a function of improvements in pulmonary hemodynamics than in systemic hemodynamics.[186–188]

To our knowledge there are no studies to define the effect of ACE inhibitors on hypoxic pulmonary vasoconstriction or gas exchange in the setting pulmonary edema or other disorders of lung function, but since pulmonary vasodilatation does occur with the administration of these agents it is possible that they could have effects similar to nitroprusside. However, in our clinical experience this has not been a problem. Clearly this would be an important area for investigation.

Inotropic Agents

This group of drugs includes two classes: digitalis glycosides and nonglycoside inotropic agents. The digitalis glycosides are derived from the foxglove plant and have been used for the treatment of CHF for more than 200 years. They still have a prominent place in the treatment of myocardial dysfunction but, their role is currently being redefined especially with discovery of the fact they have not been shown to alter the mortality of CHF while other forms of therapy have demonstrated a distinct survival advantage (i.e., ACE inhibitors, vasodilators in general, etc.). Use of the non-glycoside inotropic agents is largely confined to the treatment of the more acutely ill hospitalized patient. Either group of agents would be expected to improve pulmonary mechanics and gas exchange through improvement in cardiac output and reduction in LV filling pressure. The adverse effects on the respiratory system should be limited to perfusion redistribution leading to increased perfusion of low V/Q alveoli.

To our knowledge there are no studies to define the effect of digitalis on hypoxic pulmonary vasoconstriction or gas exchange, but the effects of two of the more commonly used non-glycoside inotropic agents, dopamine and dobutamine have been studied. In patients with CHF, dobutamine increases cardiac output and reduces CaO_2 - CVO_2, but because shunt is increased there is no change in PaO_2.[189] From studies that compare dopamine and dobutamine in a variety of animal models or clinical situations it appears that dobutamine usually produces the smaller increase in perfusion of low V/Q alveoli and shunt.[190–193] In the presence of atelectasis dobutamine may even decrease the shunt.[194]

Methylxanthines

The methylxanthines (i.e., aminophylline, theophylline, and caffeine) exert a variety of effects that should be useful in the treatment of CHF and pulmonary edema. They produce bronchodilatation, respiratory center stimulation, improved contractility of the diaphragm, and cardiovascular effects that include increased myocardial contractility and reduced vascular resistance. Indeed the classic studies of Sharp and colleagues[47] were able to demonstrate clearly beneficial effects from aminophylline in patients with CHF and pulmonary edema, which included a prompt and consistent decrease in airway resistance and a concomitant increase in pulmonary compliance. In view of the potential effects on the control of breathing and contractility of the diaphragm, it is of interest that these effects were not associated with changes in tidal volume or respiratory rate, which suggests that the primary therapeutic mechanisms included only the bronchodilator and cardiovascular effects. The improvement in VC with aminophylline in this setting reported by Heyer,[48] however, could reflect an effect on the respiratory muscles.

Bronchodilatation. Theophylline and other methylxanthines produce bronchial smooth muscle relaxation by mechanisms that are as yet unclear. There are two proposed mechanisms of action, blockage of adenosine receptors[195] and inhibition of phosphodiesterase, which results in accumulation of cyclic adenosine monophosphate (AMP) and/or cyclic guanosine monophosphate (GMP).

Respiratory Stimulation Methylxanthines stimulate the respiratory center, increase the sensitivity to CO_2 and increase the minute ventilation for any given $PaCO_2$. Aminophylline also modifies the ventilatory response to sustained hypoxia. In normal humans and laboratory animals sustained isocapnic hypoxia produces a response with accommodation to about 30% of the initial response. Pretreatment with aminophylline diminishes but does not eliminate this inhibitory effect of sustained hypoxemia.[196,197] This effect is believed to reflect central adenosine blockade.[198]

Improve Diaphragmatic Contractility and Reversal of Fatigue. Methylxanthines have been shown to increase diaphragmatic contractility[199,200] and decrease, or reverse, respiratory muscle fatigue.[201,202] Aubier et al.[203] demonstrated in dogs that theophylline increased the transdiaphragmatic pressure and diaphragmatic contractility produced by phrenic nerve stimulation in normal states and induced fatigue. The improved diaphragmatic contractility produced by methylxanthines is more pronounced during fatigue states relative to non-stressed states.

The mechanism by which these drugs augment the contractility of respiratory muscles is currently unknown but, there are a few hypotheses. The accumulation of cyclic AMP and Ca^{++} translocation could be responsible for the improved inotropic state of skeletal muscles in general.[204] Acetylcholine release at the neuromuscular junction is believed to be mediated by Ca^{++} influx in the motor nerve terminal, which can be augmented by cyclic AMP. Methylxanthines also have been demonstrated to increase the entry of Ca^{++} into muscle cells[205] and to increase the release and impede the re-uptake of

Ca^{++} by the sarcoplasmic reticulum of skeletal muscle.[206] This effect becomes very important in fatigued muscle since there is usually impaired Ca^{++} release from the sarcoplasmic reticulum during states of fatigue, which is more likely to be the cause of diminished muscle strength than is energy depletion, especially since the energy stores of fatigued muscle are usually adequate.[207]

Cardiovascular Effects. Methylxanthines also exert effects on the cardiovascular system that can accentuate the effects upon the respiratory system when used to treat CHF. They reduce PVR and increase myocardial contractility.[208,209]

Adverse Effects. Despite the many beneficial effects for the treatment of CHF and pulmonary edema, there are some potential adverse effects that must be considered before the methylxanthines are routinely applied as a panacea. These include: 1) increased heart rate with a propensity to induce tachyarrhythmias; 2) inhibition of hypoxic vasoconstriction, which could increase perfusion of low V/Q alveoli[210]; 3) agitation and seizures, 4) gastrointestinal upset; 5) multiple drug interactions and; 6) delayed drug metabolism in patients with CHF. Because if these deleterious side-effects and the low therapeutic-toxic index of methylxanthines, the use of them in the treatment of CHF and pulmonary edema is becoming less common. Although most clinical studies of this class of drug have utilized theophylline or aminophylline to evaluate their effects on the pulmonary and cardiovascular systems, a strong consideration should be given for the evaluation of caffeine in future studies instead of these more toxic agents. Caffeine has been demonstrated to have a greater potency for augmentation of contractility than the other drugs in this class.[201,211]

β-*Adrenergic Agonists*

This class of agents have been very beneficial in the treatment of asthma and bronchospasm and have been found to be beneficial in the treatment of "cardiac asthma." As the name indicates, they exert their action by binding to β-adrenergic receptors and producing the effect on these receptors that would be expected to occur with the natural β-agonists. The major hope for the use of β-adrenergic agonists has been the development of drugs with a greater specificity for the $β_2$-receptor in order to optimize bronchodilatation while minimizing $β_1$- and α-adrenergic cardiovascular effects. Despite these efforts the specificity is not yet that great and the use of β-agonists for the treatment of pulmonary dysfunction in CHF and pulmonary edema has not gained wide acceptance.

While the classic studies of Plotz[31] demonstrated significant clinical and physiologic response to subcutaneous epinephrine in patients with cardiac asthma, later studies of small airway function in patients with AMI demonstrated no benefit from the inhalation of isoproterenol,[8] suggesting that there may be a fundamental difference between cardiac asthma and small airway dysfunction in the early stages of CHF.

One interesting observation that may have future clinical relevance is that edema fluid is cleared from the alveolar space by an active transport mechanism across the alveolar epithelium, which is stimulated by β-agonists in several different mammalian species.[212,213]

Anticholinergic Agents

There are two agents in this class that are used with any frequency in the USA, atropine and ipratropium bromide. Ipratropium bromide is the only one of these that has been approved by the FDA for use as a bronchodilator, however atropine has been used in this manner for many years preceding the approval of ipratropium bromide. Because of the many systemic side-effects of atropine its use in cardiac patients is primarily in the treatment of severe and symptomatic bradycardia. Ipratropium bromide is a quaternary ammonium derivative of atropine that is poorly absorbed into the circulation and does not cross the blood-brain barrier to enter the central nervous system (CNS). The lack of CNS and cardiovascular effects make this a more attractive drug for the treatment of bronchospasm in patients with heart failure.

Ipratropium bromide is an anticholinergic/parasympatholytic drug that is a competitive inhibitor to the muscarinic acetylcholine receptors. The parasympathetic branch of the autonomic nervous system, supplied to the lungs via branches of the vagus nerve, maintains the basal tone of bronchial smooth muscle. Normally, when acetylcholine binds to muscarinic receptors it elicits bronchial smooth muscle contraction, stimulates mast cells to release a host of inflammatory mediators, and increases mucous production. Inhaled ipratropium bromide blocks these effects by competitive binding to receptors on the effector cells.[214,215] If there is increased parasympathetic input to the bronchi the effects of ipratropium bromide will be much greater.

Because the effects of anticholinergic agents form the major line of evidence implicating vagal activity in the changes in airway function in CHF, most of the therapeutic effects of these agents have already been discussed in the section of this chapter dealing with pulmonary mechanics.

Ventilatory Therapy

There are three different, but related, considerations for the application of ventilatory therapy to the management of the patient with CHF and pulmonary edema. First would be the use of mechanical ventilation to sustain life. Second would be the use of positive airway pressure to improve lung function. Third would be the use of mechanical ventilation and/or positive airway pressure to improve cardiac performance.

Ventilatory therapy to achieve these different goals can be delivered by a variety of devices including tracheal intubation, face mask, or even just a nasal appliance. The therapeutic objective should always be to use the least invasive mode consistent with the physiologic objective and patient safety. There are also a variety of different but related modes of ventilatory therapy. Positive pressure ventilation (PPV) refers to the phasic application of positive pressure to accomplish alveolar ventilation. This can be regulated either to achieve a target tidal volume, referred to as volume controlled ventilation, or to achieve a target airway pressure. When delivered via an endotracheal tube, pressure regulated PPV is referred to as pressure support ventilation (PSV). When delivered via a mask or mouthpiece it is referred to as intermittent positive pressure breathing (IPPB). Although there are subtle but important differences between the modes of PPV, these differences are beyond the scope of this discussion and PPV will be used to refer to any form of therapy with the objective of maintaining or assisting alveolar ventilation. Continuous positive airway pressure (CPAP) refers to therapy designed to achieve an increase in lung volume and intrathoracic pressure throughout the respiratory cycle. If applied to the intubated patient receiving PPV it is referred to as PEEP, positive end-expiratory pressure. Nasal CPAP, as the name implies, refers to CPAP applied via a nasal device usually for the purpose of preventing upper airway obstruction during sleep. To the extent that it accomplishes an increase in lung volume and intrathoracic pressure throughout the respiratory cycle, nasal CPAP is equivalent to CPAP, but this may not always be the case. For the purpose of this discussion CPAP refers to therapy that produces an increase lung volume and intrathoracic pressure throughout the respiratory cycle.

Mechanical Ventilation to Sustain Life

In the setting of acute cardiac failure with severely reduced cardiac output with or without pulmonary edema, mechanical ventilation can be life saving. While there are no randomized clinical studies to establish the efficacy of mechanical ventilation in cardiogenic shock, the studies of Aubier and colleagues[65,66] clearly establish that respiratory failure is the immediate preterminal event and that life can be sustained by mechanical ventilation in a canine model of cardiogenic shock. By assisting or replacing the action of the respiratory muscles PPV also reduces the work of breathing and the metabolic load on the heart.

Conventional wisdom holds that PPV reduces cardiac output[216,217] so there is appropriate concern when applying this form of treatment to a patient whose cardiac output is already severely compromised. However, the mechanism by which PPV reduces cardiac output becomes important here. This was one of the first questions addressed after the advent of cardiac catheterization in the mid 1940s. Those early studies,[217,218] and more recent studies[219–222] make it clear that the primary mechanism of reduced cardiac output with PPV involves systemic venous pooling due to increased right atrial cavitary pressure, reduced net right ventricular transmural filling pressure (P_{RVtm}), which is the difference between right ventricular cavitary pressure (P_{RV}) and pleural pressure (P_{PL}):

$$P_{RVtm} = P_{RV} - P_{PL} \qquad (3)$$

leading to decreased right ventricular end-diastolic volume (RVEDV). The increased P_{PL} also leads to reduced net left ventricular transmural filling pressure:

$$P_{LVtm} = P_{LV} - P_{PL} \qquad (4)$$

and LVEDV. Of course if P_{RA} or P_{PCW} is measured relative to body surface pressure, rather than P_{PL}, it will appear to be increased during PPV. Depending on the circumstances increased PVR due to increased alveolar pressure and lung volume may play a secondary role in the cardiac response to PPV.[221] By increasing right ventricular afterload PPV may cause deterioration of LV function due to ventricular interdependence.[223,224]

In the presence of cardiac failure or hypervolemia, filling pressures are high. Cardiac performance is determined by the flat part of the classic Starling curve and relatively insensitive to preload or end-diastolic volume. In fact under these conditions the decrease in afterload and left ventricular end-systolic volume (LVESV) during PPV may produce an increase in cardiac output.[216,225–227] The clinician should not hesitate to use mechanical ventilation in the setting of cardiogenic shock. Of course it is important that the correct diagnosis be established. The patient with reduced cardiac output due to hypovolemia, or reduced preload for any reason, will experience a further decrease in cardiac output when subjected to PPV.

Positive Airway Pressure and Lung Function

In 1909, Emerson[228] demonstrated the development of hydrostatic pulmonary edema in rabbits with high doses of epinephrine and also demonstrated that the edema could be rapidly reversed with the use of PPV. Several weeks after Emerson published his results, Barringer[229] treated a patient with CHF and pulmonary edema with PPV and noted almost complete resolution of his rales, rhonchi, and symptoms of respiratory distress with 1 hour of treatment. These results with PPV in the treatment of pulmonary edema were confirmed by several other investigators but a full understanding of this mode of therapy remained a mystery for many years. The original theories as to how positive pressure exerted its effects upon patients with decompensated CHF and pulmonary edema put forth by Emerson[228] and his contemporaries were: 1) PPV distended the lungs and drove blood out of the pulmonary vasculature and into the left heart thus alleviating pulmonary congestion and edema; 2) PPV reversed the large negative pleural pressure that was thought to occur in CHF and pulmonary edema and by doing so prevented the "negative suction" on the pulmonary capillaries and alveolar walls that promoted transudation of fluid; and 3) PPV stinted the bronchioles open thus improving alevolar ventilation and decreasing the work of breathing.[230,231]

In 1938 Barach and coworkers[108] demonstrated a marked clinical improvement with decreases in respiratory rate, increases in vital capacity, and decreases in the level of dyspnea (subjectively) in patients with CHF and pulmonary edema when treated with CPAP. Motley and the Bellevue group[216] studied the effect of PPV, tried as a last resort in four cases of severe cardiac pulmonary edema, and reported a rapid clearing of moist rales. In most patients with CHF they also demonstrated improved cardiac output as compared to normals who experienced decreased cardiac output. Sharp et al.[47] noted a consistent increase in pulmonary compliance and decrease in airway resistance in patients with decompensated CHF treated with CPAP. The explanation for the improvement in pulmonary compliance in patients with CHF treated with CPAP could be that the increase in FRC associated with positive pressure breathing places the lung on a more advantageous portion of the compliance curve[26,232] but it was also noted in these early clinical studies that the improvement in pulmonary mechanics produced by CPAP persisted after the discontinuation of CPAP suggesting that redistribution of edema fluid from the alveolar space to the peribronchial interstitial space as described by Pare et al.[111] may have occurred.

More recently it has been demonstrated that CPAP elicits a prompt improvement in gas exchange in patients with severe cardiogenic pulmonary edema. In one study, using 10 cm H_2O CPAP, a significant improvement in respiratory acidosis was demonstrated with $PaCO_2$ decreasing from 58 to 46 torr and pH increasing from 7.18 to 7.28 in the first 30 minutes of treatment, despite a 25% decrease in respiratory rate.[110] At the same time PaO_2/F_IO_2 improved from 138 ± 32 to 206 ± 126. In an earlier study, which used 30% O_2 and only 5 cm H_2O CPAP, PaO_2 increased by 8 torr during the initial 10 minutes of therapy.[109] Both studies incorporated an appropriate randomized design and in neither study did the control group experience significant improvement in gas exchange during the initial period of observation. Both studies enrolled severely ill patients that might have qualified for tracheal intubation and mechanical ventilation and the most significant finding, common to both studies, was that treatment with CPAP by face mask reduced the need for this type of invasive intervention.

Thus ventilatory therapy can improve both pulmonary mechanics and gas exchange in patients with CHF and pulmonary edema. Two of the principle mechanisms of hypoxemia, small airway closure and alveolar atelectasis, should respond to an increase in lung volume. By increasing end expiratory lung volume CPAP or PEEP will shift the tidal range of lung volumes above closing capacity and produce a decrease in hypoxemia due to low V/Q alveoli. In the patient with pulmonary edema and atelectasis due to reduced surfactant activity and alveolar instability,[101] by increasing end-expiratory transpulmonary pressure CPAP or PEEP should serve to stabilize alveoli and reduce the shunt. Even hypoxemia as the result of alveolar edema may respond to CPAP or PEEP if there is a redistribution of edema fluid from the alveolar space to the peribronchial interstitial space.[111]

Of course PaO_2 depends on both cardiac output and the shunt and therapy, which impairs cardiac output while decreasing the shunt, may not improve PaO_2 (Figure 6) and will further decrease O_2 transport to the tissues. In patients with CHF and elevated filling pressures CPAP has been shown not to impair cardiac output and to actually increase it in some cases.[226,227,233] Ventilation with PEEP should have similar effects.

Positive Airway Pressure and Cardiac Function

There are two fundamental ways in which ventilatory therapy might improve performance of the LV in patients with heart failure. First, would be a reduction in preload and end-distolic volume, and second would be a reduction in afterload and end-systolic volume.

Preload. Those who have practiced medicine for more than two decades will remember the barbaric practice of rotating tourniquets and recall the image of the dyspneic cyanotic, and sometimes edematous patient with blood pressure cuffs on three of four limbs each causing the affected extremity to become more cyanotic and more edematous. The physiologic principle was to shift blood volume from the congested central circulation to the periphery. As outlined above, ventilatory therapy with positive airway pressure can achieve this same objective while at the same time improving lung function and arterial oxygenation. With PPV or CPAP there will be an increase in mean pleural pressure and this increase in P_{PL} causes both a decrease in RVEDV and an increase in P_{RA}, relative to body surface pressure. It is this increase in P_{RA} that produces an increase both in systemic venous pressure and systemic venous volume thereby accomplishing a redistribution of blood volume just as intended with the use of rotating tourniquets. The effects of increased P_{PL} on LVEDV are less straight forward. While the immediate effect of increased P_{PL} should be to decrease the net transmural distending pressure, P_{LV} - P_{PL}, if nothing else changed, but there are other factors that change. It appears that the effect of positive airway pressure on LV afterload is the predominant factor for changes in both LVESV and LVEDV.

Afterload. The concept that LV afterload is influenced by pleural pressure can be difficult to grasp if one is used to thinking of afterload only in terms of aortic blood pressure (P_{AO}) and systemic vascular resistance. At one extreme, if pleural pressure surrounding the heart were equal to or slightly greater than P_{LV} the LV stroke volume could be ejected passively and clearly there would be no afterload. So to assess afterload under conditions of changing P_{PL} the difference between systolic P_{LV} and P_{PL} becomes the critical determinant of afterload. If there is no gradient across the aortic valve P_{AO} and systolic P_{LV} are equal and it is convenient to express afterload as P_{AO} - P_{PL}. Normally, changes in P_{PL} are small relative to P_{AO} and little error is introduced by ignoring the pleural pressure, but with large increase in P_{PL}, which occurs during the Valsalva maneuver (a maximal expiratory effort at total lung capacity with the glottis closed), or with the large negative swing in P_{PL}, which occurs during the Mueller maneuver (a maximal inspiratory effort at residual volume with the glottis closed), it is necessary to take P_{PL} into consideration to account for the observed changes in left ventricular volume, ejection fraction, and the velocity of fiber shortening.[223]

When dyspneic patients with increased airway resistance and decreased lung compliance are struggling to get their breath, similar extremes of pleural pressure swings can occur and it becomes important to include pleural pressure changes in the development of a strategy to optimize cardiac performance. It has been demonstrated that large negative swings in pleural pressure can aggravate regional abnormalities in myocardial function due to ischemic heart disease.[234]

Summary

In this chapter, we have sought to present CHF from a pulmonary perspective emphasizing key concepts that impact on the assessment and management of patients. These include the following:

(1) The evolution of pulmonary vascular congestion and edema occurs in stages—each with distinct clinical characteristics.
(2) There is good correlation between vascular pressures and measures of pulmonary mechanics and gas exchange. Such a relationship does not consistently hold for radiographic manifestations.

(3) Airway obstruction in compensated as well as decompensated states is becoming increasingly recognized. This has implications for management in both the acute and chronic settings.

(4) Respiratory muscle function may be impaired contributing to symptoms and potentially to respiratory failure when there is acute decompensation.

(5) Alterations in gas exchange are influenced by many factors including lung volume changes, pulmonary blood flow redistribution, cardiac output, and acid-base status. Although the significance of these factors varies among patients, the identification of the predominant pathophysiologic mechanisms in a given patient may be essential for optimal management.

(6) Despite the plethora of therapeutic options, the basic principles of reductions in preload and afterload and augmentation of cardiac output still apply. The use of oxygen, various pharmacologic agents, and ventilatory support—all of which have circulatory as well as respiratory actions—may each have some role in a given patient's medical regimen.

References

1. Staub NC, Nagano H, Pearce ML. Pulmonary edema in dogs, especially the sequence of fluid accumulation in lungs. J Appl Physiol 1967;22:227–240.
2. Conhaim RL. Airway level at which edema liquid enters the air space of isolated dog lungs. J Appl Physiol 1989;67:2234–2242.
3. Bachofen H, Schurch S, Weibel ER. Experimental hydrostatic pulmonary edema in rabbit lungs. Barrier lesions. Am Rev Respir Dis 1993;147:997–1004.
4. Rippe B, Townsley M, Thigpen J, et al. Effects of vascular pressure on the pulmonary microvasculature in isolated dog lungs. J Appl Physiol 1984;57:233–239.
5. Tsukimoto K, Mathieu-Costello O, Prediletto R, et al. Ultrastructural appearances of pulmonary capillaries at high transmural pressures. J Appl Physiol 1991;71:573–582.
6. Peabody FW, Wentworth JA. Clinical studies of the respiration. IV. The vital capacity of the lungs and its relation to dyspnea. Arch Intern Med 1917;20:443–467.
7. Kannel WB, Seidman JM, Fercho W, et al. Vital capacity and congestive heart failure. The Framingham study. Circulation 1974;49:1160–1166.
8. Interiano B, Hyde RW, Hodges M, et al. Interrelation between alterations in pulmonary mechanics and hemodynamics in acute myocardial infarction. J Clin Invest 1973;52:1994–2006.
9. Hales CA, Kazemi H. Clinical significance of pulmonary function tests. Pulmonary function after uncomplicated myocardial infarction. Chest 1977;72:350–358.
10. Gray BA, Hyde RW, Hodges M, et al. Alterations in lung volume and pulmonary function in relation to hemodynamic changes in acute myocardial infarction. Circulation 1979;59:551–559.

11. Muir AL, Flenley DC, Kirby BJ, et al. Cardiorespiratory effects of rapid saline infusion in normal man. J Appl Physiol 1975;38:786–775.
12. Giuntini C, Maseri A, Bianchi R. Pulmonary vascular distensibility and lung compliance as modified by dextran infusion and subsequent atropine injection in normal subjects. J Clin Invest 1966;45:1770–1789.
13. Ries AL, Gregoratos G, Friedman PJ, et al. Pulmonary function tests in the detection of left heart failure: correlation with pulmonary artery wedge pressure. Respiration 1986;49:241–250.
14. Peters JP Jr, Barr DP. Studies of the respiratory mechanism in cardiac dyspnea: II. A note on the effective lung volume in cardiac dyspnea. Am J Physiol 1920;54:335–344.
15. Frank NR, Lyons HA, Siebens AA, et al. Pulmonary compliance in patients with cardiac disease. Am J Med 1957;22:516–523.
16. Goldman HI, Becklake MR. Respiratory Function Tests: normal values at median altitudes and the prediction of normal results. Am Rev Tuberc Pulm Dis 1959;79:457–467.
17. Demedts M, Sniderman A, Utz G, et al. Lung volumes including closing volume, and arterial boood gas measurements in acute ischaemic left heart failure. Bull Physiopathol Respir (Nancy) 1974;10:11–25.
18. Light RW, George RB. Serial pulmonary function in patients with acute heart failure. Arch Intern Med 1983;143:429–433.
19. Woolcock AJ, Rebuck AS, Cade JF, et al. Lung volume changes in asthma measured concurrently by two methods. Am Rev Respir Dis 1971;104:703–709.
20. Goeree GW, Coates G, Powles AC, et al. Mechanisms of changes in nitrogen washout and lung volumes after saline infusion in humans. Am Rev Respir Dis 1987;136:824–828.
21. Gray BA, McCaffree DR, Sivak ED, et al. Effect of pulmonary vascular engorgement on respiratory mechanics in the dog. J Appl Physiol 1978;45:119–127.
22. Saxton GA, Rabinowitz M, Dexter L, et al. The relationship of pulmonary compliance to pulmonary vascular pressures in patients with heart disease. J Clin Invest 1956;35:611–617.
23. Bondurant S, Hickam JB, Isley JK. Pulmonary and circulatory effects of acute pulmonary vascular engorgement in normal subjects. J Clin Invest 1957;36: 59–66.
24. Bondurant S, Mead J, Cook CD. A re-evaluation of effects of acute central congestion on pulmonary compliance in normal subjects. J Appl Physiol 1960;15: 875– 877.
25. Noble WH, Kay JC, Obdrzalek J. Lung mechanics in hypervolemic pulmonary edema. J Appl Physiol 1975;38:681–687.
26. Sharp JT, Griffith GT, Bunnell IL, et al. Ventilatory mechanics in pulmonary edema in man. J Clin Invest 1958;37:111–117.
27. Spencer H. Pathology of the lung, Third Ed. Oxford, Pergamon Press, 1977, pp. 621–622.
28. Pai U, McMahon J, Tomashefski JF Jr. Mineralizing pulmonary elastosis in chronic cardiac failure. "Endogenous pneumoconiosis" revisited. Am J Clin Pathol 1994;101:22–28.
29. Estenne M, Yernault JC, DeTroyer A. Mechanism of relief of dyspnea after thoracocentesis in patients with large pleural effusions. Am J Med 1983;74:813–819.
30. Snashall PD, Chung KF. Airway obstruction and bronchial hyperresponsiveness in left ventricular failure and mitral stenosis. Am Rev Respir Dis 1991;144: 945–956.
31. Plotz M. Bronchial spasm in cardiac asthma. Ann Intern Med 1947;26:521–525.

32. Cosby RS, Stowell EC, Hartwig WR, et al. Pulmonary function in left ventricular failure, including cardiac asthma. Circulation 1957;15:492–501.
33. Hogg JC, Agarawal JB, Gardiner AJ, et al. Distribution of airway resistance with developing pulmonary edema in dogs. J Appl Physiol 1972;32:20–24.
34. Ishii M, Matsumoto N, Fuyuki T, et al. Effects of hemodynamic edema formation on peripheral vs. central airway mechanics. J Appl Physiol 1985;59: 1578–1584.
35. Faridy EE, Permutt S. Surface forces and airway obstruction. J Appl Physiol 1971;30:319–321.
36. Macklem PT, Mead J. Resistance of central and peripheral airways measured by a retrograde catheter. J Appl Physiol 1967;22:395–401.
37. Milic-Emili J, Ruff F. Effects of pulmonary congestion and edema on the small airways. Bull Physiopathol Respir (Nancy) 1971;7:1181–1196.
38. Iliff LD, Greene RE, Hughes JM. Effect of interstitial edema on distribution of ventilation and perfusion in isolated lung. J Appl Physiol 1972;33:462–467.
39. Michel RP, Zocchi L, Rossi A, et al. Does interstitial lung edema compress airways and arteries? A morphometric study. J Appl Physiol 1987;62;108–115.
40. Kappagoda CT, Man GC, Teo KK. Behaviour of canine pulmonary vagal afferent receptors during sustained acute pulmonary venous pressure elevation. J Physiol (Lond) 1987;394:249–265.
41. Roberts AM, Bhattacharya J, Schultz HD, et al. Stimulation of pulmonary vagal afferent C-fibers by lung edema in dogs. Circulation Res 1986;58:512–522.
42. Chung KF, Keyes SJ, Morgan BM, et al. Mechanisms of airway narrowing in acute pulmonary oedema in dogs: influence of the vagus and lung volume. Clin Sci 1983;65:289–296.
43. Pepine CJ, Wiener L. Relationship of anginal symptoms to lung mechanics during myocardial ischemia. Circulation 1972;46:863–869.
44. Hales CA, Kazemi H. Small-airways function in myocardial infarction. N Engl J Med 1974;290:761–765.
45. Rolla G, Bucca C, Polizzi S, et al. Site of airway obstruction after rapid saline infusion in healthy subjects. Respiration 1983;44:90–96.
46. Collins JV, Clark TJ, Brown DJ. Airway function in healthy subjects and patients with left heart disease. Clin Sci 1975;49:217–228.
47. Sharp JT, Bunnell IL, Griffith GT, et al. The effects of therapy on pulmonary mechanics in human pulmonary edema. J Clin Invest 1961;40:665–672.
48. Heyer HE. Abnormalities of the respiratory pattern in patients with cardiac dyspnea. Am Heart J 1946; 32:457–467.
49. Rolla G, Bucca C, Brussino L, et al. Bronchodilating effect of ipratropium bromide in heart failure. Eur Respir J 1993;6:1492–1495.
50. Cabanes LR, Weber SN, Matron R, et al. Bronchial hyperresponsiveness to methacholine in patients with impaired left ventricular function. N Engl J Med 1989;320:1317–1322.
51. Cabanes L, Costes F, Weber S, et al. Improvement in exercise performance by inhalation of methoxamine in patients with impaired left ventricular function. N Engl J Med 1992;326:1661–1665.
52. Brunnee T, Graf K, Kastens B, et al. Bronchial hyperreactivity in patients with moderate pulmonary circulation overload. Chest 1993;103:1477–1481.
53. Sasaki F, Ishizaki T, Mifune J, et al. Bronchial hyperresponsiveness in patients with chronic congestive heart failure. Chest 1990;97:534–538.
54. Pison C, Malo JL, Rouleau JL, et al. Bronchial hyperresponsiveness to inhaled methacholine in subjects with chronic left heart failure at a time of exacerbation and after increasing diuretic therapy. Chest 1989;96:230–235.

55. Eichacker PQ, Seidelman MJ, Rothstein MS, et al. Methacholine bronchial reactivity testing in patients with chronic congestive heart failure. Chest 1988;93: 336– 338.
56. Seibert AF, Allison RC, Bryars CH, et al. Normal airway responsiveness to methacholine in cardiac asthma. Am Rev Respir Dis 1989;140:1805–1806.
57. Kikuchi R, Sekizawa K, Sasaki H, et al. Effects of pulmonary congestion on airway reactivity to histamine aerosol in dogs. J Appl Physiol 1984;57:1640–1647.
58. Lockhart A, Dinh-Xuan AT, Regnard J, et al. Effect of airway blood flow on airflow. Am Rev Respir Dis 1992;146:S19–23.
59. Hammond MD, Bauer KA, Sharp JT, et al. Respiratory muscle strength in congestive heart failure. Chest 1990;98:1091–1094.
60. Ambrosino N, Opasich C, Crotti P, et al. Breathing pattern, ventilatory drive and respiratory muscle strength in patients with chronic heart failure. Eur Respir J 1994;7:17–22.
61. Nishimura Y, Maeda H, Tanaka K, et al. Respiratory muscle strength and hemodynamics in chronic heart failure. Chest 1994;105:355–359.
62. Mancini DM, Henson D, LaManca J, et al. Respiratory muscle function and dyspnea in patients with chronic congestive heart failure. Circulation 1992;86: 909–918.
63. McParland C, Krishnan B, Wang Y, et al. Inspiratory muscle weakness and dyspnea in chronic heart failure. Am Rev Respir Dis 1992;146:467–472.
64. Mancini DM, Ferraro N, Nazzaro D, et al. Respiratory muscle deoxygenation during exercise in patients with heart failure demonstrated with near-infrared spectroscopy. J Am Coll Cardiol 1991;18:492–498.
65. Aubier M, Trippenbach T, Roussos C. Respiratory muscle fatigue during cardiogenic shock. J Appl Physiol 1981;51:499–508.
66. Aubier M, Viires N, Syllie G, et al. Respiratory muscle contribution to lactic acidosis in low cardiac output. Am Rev Respir Dis 1982;126:648–652.
67. Schreiner BF Jr, Murphy GW, Kramer DH, et al. The pathophysiology of pulmonary congestion. Prog Cardiovasc Dis 1971;14:57–80.
68. Harris P, Heath D. The human pulmonary circulation: Its form and function in health and disease. London, Churchill Livingstone, 1977, pp. 348–350.
69. Dollery CT, West JB. Regional uptake of radioactive oxygen, carbon monoxide and carbon dioxide in the lungs of patients with mitral stenosis. Circ Res 1960;8:765–771.
70. Friedman WF, Braunwald E. Alterations in regional pulmonary blood flow in mitral valve disease studied by radioisotope scanning. A simple nontraumatic technique for estimation of left atrial pressure. Circulation 1966;34:363–376.
71. Simon M. The pulmonary vessels in incipient left ventricular decompensation: Radiologic observations. Circulation 1961;24:185–190.
72. Turner AF, Lau FY, Jacobson G. A method for the estimation of pulmonary venous and arterial pressures from the routine chest roentgenogram. Am J Roentgenol Radium Ther Nucl Med 1972;116:97–106.
73. Surette GD, Muir AL, Hogg JC, et al. Roentgenographic study of blood flow redistribution in acute pulmonary edema in dogs. Invest Radiol 1975;10:109–114.
74. West JB, Dollery CT, Heard BE. Increased pulmonary vascular resistance in the dependent lung zone of the isolated dog lung caused by perivascular edema. Circ Res 1965;17:191–206.
75. Hughes JM, Glazier JB, Maloney JE, et al. Effect of extra-alveolar vessels on distribution of blood flow in the dog lung. J Appl Physiol 1968;25:701–712.

76. Hughes JM, Glazier JB, Maloney JE, et al. Effect of lung volume on the distribution of pulmonary blood flow in man. Respir Physiol 1968;4:58–72.

77. West JB, Dollery CT, Naimark A. Distribution of blood flow in isolated lung; relation to vascular and alveolar pressures. J Appl Physiol 1964;19:713–724.

78. Hughes JM, Glazier JB, Rosenzweig DY, et al. Factors determining the distribution of pulmonary blood flow in patients with raised pulmonary venous pressure. Clin Sci 1969;37:847–858.

79. Muir AL, Hall DL, Despas P, et al. Distribution of blood flow in the lungs in acute pulmonary edema in dogs. J Appl Physiol 1972;33:763–769.

80. Muir AL, Hogg JC, Naimark A, et al. Effect of alveolar liquid on distribution of blood flow in dogs lungs. J Appl Physiol 1975;39:885–890.

81. Tsang JY, Baile EM, Hogg JC. Relationship between regional pulmonary edema and blood flow. J Appl Physiol 1986;60:449–457.

82. Ali J, Wood LD. Factors affecting perfusion distribution in canine oleic acid pulmonary edema. J Appl Physiol 1986;60:1498–1503.

83. Carlile PV, Hagan SF, Gray BA. Perfusion distribution and lung thermal volume in canine hydrochloric acid aspiration. J Appl Physiol 1988;65:750–759.

84. Montaner JSG, Tsang J, Evans KG, et al. Alveolar epithelial damage: A critical difference between high pressure and oleic acid-induced low pressure pulmonary edema. J Clin Invest 1986;77:1786–1796.

85. Ghignone M, Girling L, Prewitt RM. Effects of vasodilators on canine cardiopulmonary function when a decrease in cardiac output complicates an increase in right ventricular afterload. Am Rev Respir Dis 1985;131:527–530.

86. Adnot S, Radermacher P, Andrivet P, et al. Effects of sodium-nitroprusside and urapidil on gas exchange and ventilation-perfusion relationships in patients with congestive heart failure. Eur Respir J 1991;4:69–75.

87. Prewitt RM, Wood LD. Effect of sodium nitroprusside on cardiovascular function and pulmonary shunt in canine oleic acid pulmonary edema. Anesthesiology 1981;55:537–541.

88. Palmaz JC, Barnett CA, Reich SB, et al. Reverse ventilation—perfusion mismatch. Clin Nucl Med 1984;9:6–9.

89. Brimioulle S, Lejeune P, Vachiery JL, et al. Effects of acidosis and alkalosis on hypoxic pulmonary vasoconstriction in dogs. Am J Physiol 1990;258:H347–53.

90. Fike CD, Hansen TN. The effect of alkalosis on hypoxia-induced pulmonary vasoconstriction in lungs of newborn rabbits. Pediatr Res 1989;25:383–388.

91. Schreiber MD, Heymann MA, Soifer SJ. Increased arterial pH, not decreased PaCO2, attenuates hypoxia-induced pulmonary vasoconstriction in newborn lambs. Pediatr Res 1986;20:113–117.

92. McHugh TJ, Forrester JS, Adler L, et al. Pulmonary vascular congestion in acute myocardial infarction: hemodynamic and radiologic correlations. Ann Intern Med 1972;76:29–33.

93. Chakko S, Woska D, Martinez H, et al. Clinical, radiographic, and hemodynamic correlations in chronic congestive heart failure: conflicting results may lead to inappropriate care. Am J Med 1991;90:353–359.

94. Nixon PG. Pulmonary oedema with low left ventricular diastolic pressure in acute myocardial infarction. Lancet 1968;2:146–147.

95. Slutsky RA, Higgins CB. Intravascular and extravascular pulmonary fluid volumes II. Response to rapid increases in left atrial pressure and the theoretical implications for pulmonary radiographic and radionuclide imaging. Invest Radiol 1983;18:33–39.

96. Schober OH, Meyer GJ, Bossaller C, et al. Quantitative determination of regional extravascular lung water and regional blood volume in congestive heart failure. Eur J Nucl Med 1985;10:17–24.
97. Rosenow EC III, Harrison CE Jr. Congestive heart failure masquerading as primary pulmonary disease. Chest 1970;58:28–36.
98. Leith DE, Mead J. Mechanisms determining residual volume of the lungs in normal subjects. J Appl Physiol 1967;23:221–227.
99. Craig DB, Wahba WM, Don HF, et al. "Closing volume" and its relationship to gas exchange in seated and supine positions. J Appl Physiol 1971;31:717–721.
100. Jones JG, Lemen R, Graf PD. Changes in airway calibre following pulmonary venous congestion. Br J Anaesth 1978;50:743–752.
101. Said SI, Avery ME, Davis RK, et al. Pulmonary surface activity in induced pulmonary edema. J Clin Invest 1965;44:458–464.
102. Dantzker DR, Wagner PD, West JB. Instability of lung units with low Va/Q ratios during O2 breathing. J Appl Physiol 1975;83:886–895.
103. Sutherland PW, Cade JF, Pain MC. Pulmonary extravascular fluid volume and hypoxaemia in myocardial infarction. Aust N Z J Med 1971;1:141–145.
104. Higgs BE. Factors influencing pulmonary gas exchange during the acute stages of myocardial infarction. Clin Sci 1968;35:115–122.
105. Valencia A, Burgess JH. Arterial hypoxemia following acute myocardial infarction. Circulation 1969;40:641–652.
106. Scheinman MM, Evans GT. Right to left shunt in patients with acute myocardial infarction. A proposed mechanism. Am J Cardiol 1972;29:757–766.
107. Barach AL, Martin J, Eckman M. Positive pressure respiration and its application to the treatment of acute pulmonary edema and respiratory obstruction. Proc Am Soc Clin Invest 1937;26:664.
108. Barach AL, Martin J, Eckman M. Positive pressure respiration and its application to the treatment of acute pulmonary edema. Ann Intern Med 1938;12:754–795.
109. Rasanen J, Heikkila J, Downs J, et al. Continuous positive airway pressure by face mask in acute cardiogenic pulmonary edema. Am J Cardiol 1985; 55:296–300.
110. Bersten AD, Holt AW, Vedig AE, et al. Treatment of severe cardiogenic pulmonary edema with continuous positive airway pressure delivered by face mask. N Engl J Med 1991;325:1825–1830.
111. Pare PD, Warriner B, Baile EM, et al. Redistribution of pulmonary extravascular water with positive end-expiratory pressure in canine pulmonary edema. Am Rev Respir Dis 1983;127:590–593.
112. Pande JN, Gupta SP, Guleria JS. Clinical significance of the measurement of membrane diffusing capacity and pulmonary capillary blood volume. Respiration 1975;32:317–324.
113. Siegel JL, Miller A, Brown LK, et al. Pulmonary diffusing capacity in left ventricular dysfunction. Chest 1990;98:550–553.
114. Palmer WH, Gee JBL, Mills FC, et al. Disturbances of pulmonary function in mitral valve disease. Canad M A J 1963;89:744–750.
115. Rhodes KM, Evemy K, Nariman S, et al. Relation between severity of mitral valve disease and results of routine lung function tests in non-smokers. Thorax 1982;37:751–755.
116. MacKenzie GJ, Flenley DC, Taylor SH, et al. Circulatory and respiratory studies in myocardial infarction and cardiogenic shock. Lancet 1964;2:825–832.

117. Davidson RM, Ramo BW, Wallace AG, et al. Blood-gas and hemodynamic responses to oxygen in acute myocardial infarction. Circulation 1973;47: 704–711.
118. Fillmore SJ, Shapiro M, Killip T. Arterial oxygen tension in acute myocardial infarction. Serial analysis of clinical state and blood gas changes. Am Heart J 1970;79:620–629.
119. Sukumalchantra Y, Danzig R, Levy SE, et al. The mechanism of arterial hypoxemia in acute myocardial infarction. Circulation 1970;41:641–650.
120. Lynch JP, Mhyre JG, Dantzker DR. Influence of cardiac output on intrapulmonary shunt. J Appl Physiol 1979;46:315–321.
121. Westbrook JL, Sykes MK. Peroperative arterial hypoxaemia. The interaction between intrapulmonary shunt and cardiac output. A computer model. Anaesthesia 1992;47:307–310.
122. Dantzker DR. The influence of cardiovascular function on gas exchange. Clin Chest Med 1983;4:149–159.
123. Smith G, Cheney FW, Winter PM. Proceedings: The contribution of mixed venous oxygenation to the change in Qs-Qt that occurs with change in cardiac output. Br J Anaesth 1973;45:1230–1231.
124. Breen PH, Schumacker PT, Hedenstierna G, et al. How does increased cardiac output increase shunt in pulmonary edema? J Appl Physiol 1982;53:1273–1280.
125. Breen PH, Schumacker PT, Sandoval J, et al. Increased cardiac output increases shunt: role of pulmonary edema and perfusion. J Appl Physiol 1985;59: 1313–1321.
126. Benumof JL, Pirlo AS, Johanson I, et al. Interaction of PvO_2 with PAO_2 on hypoxic pulmonary vasoconstriction. J Appl Physiol 1981;51:871–874.
127. Fillmore SJ, Guimaraes AC, Scheidt SS, et al. Blood-gas changes and pulmonary hemodynamics following acute myocardial infarction. Circulation 1972;45:583–591.
128. Tattersfield AE, McNicol MW, Sillett RW. Relationship between haemodynamic and respiratory function in patients with myocardial infarction and left ventricular failure. Clin Sci 1972;42:751–768 .
129. Lassers BW, George M, Anderton JL, et al. Left ventricular failure in acute myocardial infarction. Am J Cardiol 1970;25:511–522.
130. Friedman BL, Macias JJ, Yu PN. Pulmonary function studies in patients with mitral stenosis. Am Rev Tuberc 1959;79:265–272.
131. Avery WG, Samet P, Sackner MA. The acidosis of pulmonary edema. Am J Med 1970;48:320–324.
132. Aberman A, Fulop M: The metabolic and respiratory acidosis of acute pulmonary edema. Ann Intern Med 1972;76:173–184.
133. O'Donovan R, McGowan JA, Lupinacci L, et al. Acid-base disturbances in cardiogenic pulmonary edema. Nephron 1991;57:416–420.
134. Saunders KB. Physiological dead space in left ventricular failure. Clin Sci 1966;31:145–151.
135. McNicol MW, Kirby BJ, Bhools KD, et al. Pulmonary function in acute myocardial infarction. Br Med J 1965;2:1270–1273.
136. Pain MC, Stannard M, Sloman G. Disturbances of pulmonary function after acute myocardial infarction. Br Med J 1967;2:591–594.
137. Wilson JR, Mancini DM. Factors contributing to the exercise limitation of heart failure. J Am Coll Cardiol 1993;22:93A–98A.

138. Sullivan MJ, Higginbotham MB, Cobb FR. Increased exercise ventilation in patients with chronic heart failure: intact ventilatory control despite hemodynamic and pulmonary abnormalities. Circulation 1988;77:552–559.
139. Weber KT, Kinasewitz GT, Janicki JS, et al. Oxygen utilization and ventilation during exercise in patients with chronic cardiac failure. Circulation 1982;65:1213–1223.
140. Sovijarvi AR, Naveri H, Leinonen H. Ineffective ventilation during exercise in patients with chronic congestive heart failure. Clin Physiol 1992;12:309–408.
141. Wada O, Asanoi H, Miyagi K, et a. Importance of abnormal lung perfusion in excessive exercise ventilation in chronic heart failure. Am Heart J 1993;125:790–798.
142. Brimioulle S, Vachiery JL, Lejeune P, et al. Acid-base status affects gas exchange in canine oleic acid pulmonary edema. Am J Physiol 1991;260:H1080–6.
143. Domino KB, Lu Y, Eisenstein BL, et al. Hypocapnia worsens arterial blood oxygenation and increases VA/Q heterogeneity in canine pulmonary edema. Anesthesiology 1993;78:91–99.
144. Brimioulle S, Kahn RJ. Effects of metabolic alkalosis on pulmonary gas exchange. Am Rev Respir Dis 1990;141:1185–1189.
145. Lichtman MA, Cohen J, Young JA, et al. The relationships between arterial oxygen flow rate, oxygen binding by hemoglobin, and oxygen utilization after myocardial infarction. J Clin Invest 1974;54:501–513.
146. Daniel A, Cohen J, Lichtman MA, et al. The relationships among arterial oxygen flow rate, oxygen binding by hemoglobin, and oxygen utilization in chronic cardiac decompensation. J Lab Clin Med 1978;91:635–649.
147. Valeri CR, Fortier NL. Red-cell 2,3-diphosphoglycerate and creatine levels in patients with red-cell mass deficits or with cardiopulmonary insufficiency. N Engl J Med 1969;281:1452–1455.
148. Bellingham AJ, Detter JC, Lenfant C. Regulatory mechanisms of hemoglobin oxygen affinity in acidosis and alkalosis. J Clin Invest 1971;50:700–706.
149. Vismara LA, Leaman DM, Zelis R. The effects of morphine on venous tone in patients with acute pulmonary edema. Circulation 1976;54:335–337.
150. Leaman DM, Levenson L, Zelis R, et al. Effect of morphine on splanchnic blood flow. Br Heart J 1978;40:569–571.
151. Flaim SF, Vismara LA, Zelis R. The effects of morphine on isolated cutaneous canine vascular smooth muscle. Res Common Chem Pathol Pharmacol 1977;16:191–194.
152. Timmis AD, Rothman MT, Henderson MA, et al. Haemodynamic effects of intravenous morphine in patients with acute myocardial infarction complicated by severe left ventricular failure. Br Med J 1980;280:980–982.
153. Grossman W, McLaurin LP, Rolett EL. Alterations in left ventricular relaxation and diastolic compliance in congestive cardiomyopathy. Cardiovasc Res 1979;13:514–522.
154. Pierpont GL, DeMaster EG, Cohn JN. Regional differences in adrenergic function within the left ventricle. Am J Physiol 1984;246:H824–9.
155. Pierpoint GL, Francis GS, DeMaster EG, et al. Heterogeneous myocardial catecholamine concentrations in patients with congestive heart failure. Am J Cardiol 1987;60:316–321.
156. Blaustein AS, Gaasch WH. Myocardial relaxation. VI. Effects of beta-adrenergic tone and asynchrony on LV relaxation rate. Am J Physiol 1983;244:H417–22.

157. Siwadlowski W, Aravanis C, Worthen M, et al. Mechanism of adrenalin pulmonary edema and its prevention by narcotics and autonomic blockers. Chest 1970;57:554–557.
158. Biagi RW, Bapat BN. Frusemide in acute pulmonary oedema. Lancet 1967;1:849.
159. Dikshit K, Vyden JK, Forrester JS, et al. Renal and extrarenal hemodynamic effects of furosemide in congestive heart failure after acute myocardial infarction. N Engl J Med 1973;288:1087–1090.
160. Austin SM, Schreiner BF, Kramer DH, et al. The acute hemodynamic effects of ethacrynic acid and furosemide in patients with chronic postcapillary pulmonary hypertension. Circulation 1976;53:364–369.
161. Johnston GD, Nicholls DP, Leahey WJ. The dose-response characteristics of the acute non-diuretic peripheral vascular effects of frusemide in normal subjects. Br J Clin Pharmacol 1984;18:75–81.
162. Silber S, Vogler AC, Spiegelsberger F, et al. The insufficient nitrate response: patients' characterization and response to beta and calcium blockade. Eur Heart J 1988;9(Suppl A):125–134.
163. Biddle TL, Yu PN. Effect of furosemide on hemodynamics and lung water in acute pulmonary edema secondary to myocardial infarction. Am J Cardiol 1979;43:86–90.
164. Iff HW, Flenley DC. Blood-gas exchange after frusemide in acute pulmonary oedema. Lancet 1971;1:616–618.
165. Tattersfield AE, McNicol MW. Frusemide and pulmonary oedema. Lancet 1971;1:911.
166. Evan CL, Matsuoka Y. The effects of various mechanical conditions on the gaseous metabolism and efficiency of the mammalian heart. J Physiol (Lond) 1915;49:378–405.
167. Sarnoff SJ, Braunwald E, Welch GH. Hemodynamic determinants of oxygen consumption of the heart with special reference to the tension time index. Am J Physiol 1958;192:148–156.
168. Rodbard S, Williams CB, Rodbard D, et al. Myocardial tension and oxygen uptake. Circulation Res 1964;14:139–149.
169. Graham TP, Covell JW, Sonnenblick EH, et al. Control of myocardial oxygen consumption: relative influence of contractile state and tension development. J Clin Invest 1968;47:375–385.
170. Krantz JC, Jr. Action and nomenclature of nitroglycerin and nitrate esters. Am J Cardiol 1972;29:436–438.
171. Johnson JB, Gross JF, Hale H. Effects of sublingual administration of nitroglycerin on pulmonary artery pressure in patients with failure of the left ventricle. N Engl J Med 1957;257:1114–1117.
172. Bussmann WD, Schupp D: Effect of sublingual nitroglycerin in emergency treatment of severe pulmonary edema. Am J Cardiol 1978;41:931–936.
173. Franciosa JA, Limas CJ, Guiha NH, et al. Improved left ventricular function during nitroprusside infusion in acute myocardial infarction. Lancet 1972;1:650–654.
174. Guiha NH, Cohn JN, Mikulic E, et al. Treatment of refractory heart failure with infusion of nitroprusside. N Engl J Med 1974;291:587–592.
175. Miller RR, Vismara LA, Williams DO, et al. Pharmacological mechanisms for left ventricular unloading in clinical congestive heart failure. Differential effects of nitroprusside, phentolamine, and nitroglycerin on cardiac function and peripheral circulation. Circ Res 1976;39:127–133.

176. Sivak ED, Gray BA, McCurdy HT, et al. Pulmonary vascular response to nitroprusside in dogs. Circ Res 1979;45:360–365.
177. Kadowitz PJ, Nandiwada P, Gruetter CA, et al. Pulmonary vasodilator responses to nitroprusside and nitroglycerin in the dog. J Clin Invest 1981;67:893–902.
178. D'Oliveira M, Sykes MK, Chakrabarti MK, et al. Depression of hypoxic pulmonary vasoconstriction by sodium nitroprusside and nitroglycerine. Br J Anaesth 1981;53:11–18.
179. Hales CA, Westphal D. Hypoxemia following the administration of sublingual nitroglycerin. Am J Med 1978;65:911–918.
180. Annest SJ, Gottlieb ME, Rhodes GR, et al. Nitroprusside and nitroglycerine in patients with posttraumatic pulmonary failure. J Trauma 1981;21:1029–1031.
181. Ghignone M, Girling L, Prewitt RM. Effects of hydralazine on cardiopulmonary function in canine low-pressure pulmonary edema. Anesthesiology 1983;59:187–190.
182. Ader R, Chatterjee K, Ports T, et al. Immediate and sustained hemodynamic and clinical improvement in chronic heart failure by an oral angiotension-converting enzyme inhibitor. Circulation 1980;61:931–937.
183. Dzau VJ, Colucci WS, Williams GH, et al. Sustained effectiveness of converting-enzyme inhibition in patients with severe congestive heart failure. N Engl J Med 1980;302:1373–1379.
184. CONSENSUS TS. Effects of enalapril on mortality in severe congestive heart failure. Results of the Cooperative North Scandinavian Enalapril Survival Study (CONSENSUS). The CONSENSUS Trial Study Group. N Engl J Med 1987;316:1429–1435.
185. SOLVD. Effect of enalapril on survival in patients with reduced left ventricular ejection fractions and congestive heart failure. The SOLVD Investigators. N Engl J Med 1991;325:293–302.
186. Pelliccia F, Borghi A, Ruggeri A, et al. Changes in pulmonary hemodynamics predict benefits in exercise capacity after ACE inhibition in patients with mild to moderate congestive heart failure. Clin Cardiol 1993;16:607–612.
187. Franciosa JA, Baker BJ, Seth L. Pulmonary versus systemic hemodynamics in determining exercise capacity of patients with chronic left ventricular failure. Am Heart J 1985;110:807–813.
188. Packer M, Lee WH, Medina N, et al. Hemodynamic and clinical significance of the pulmonary vascular response to long-term captopril therapy in patients with severe chronic heart failure. J Am Coll Cardiol 1985;6:635–645.
189. Erlemeier HH, Kupper W, Bleifeld W. Effect of dobutamine on pulmonary gas exchange in patients with severe heart failure. Eur Heart J 1992;13:1545–1548.
190. Molloy DW, Ducas J, Dobson K, et al. Hemodynamic management in clinical acute hypoxemic respiratory failure. Dopamine vs dobutamine. Chest 1986;89:636–640.
191. Light RB, Ali J, Breen P, et al. The pulmonary vascular effects of dopamine, dobutamine, and isoproterenol in unilobar pulmonary edema in dogs. J Surg Res 1988;44:26–35.
192. Nomoto Y, Kawamura M. Pulmonary gas exchange effects by nitroglycerin, dopamine and dobutamine during one-lung ventilation in man. Can J Anaesth 1989;36:273–277.
193. Rennotte MT, Reynaert M, Clerbaux T, et al. Effects of two inotropic drugs, dopamine and dobutamine, on pulmonary gas exchange in artificially ventilated patients. Intensive Care Med 1989;15:160–165.

194. Mathru M, Dries DJ, Kanuri D, et al. Effect of cardiac output on gas exchange in one-lung atelectasis. Chest 1990;97:1121–1124.
195. Fredholm BB, Persson CG. Xanthine derivatives as adenosine receptor antagonists. Eur J Pharmacol 1982;81:673–676.
196. Easton PA, Anthonisen NR. Ventilatory response to sustained hypoxia after pretreatment with aminophylline. J Appl Physiol 1988;64:1445–1450.
197. Georgopoulos D, Holtby SG, Berezanski D, et al. Aminophylline effects on ventilatory response to hypoxia and hyperoxia in normal adults. J Appl Physiol 1989;67:1150–1156.
198. Long WQ, Anthonisen NR. Aminophylline partially blocks ventilatory depression with hypoxia in the awake cat. Can J Physiol Pharmacol 1994;72:673–678.
199. Aubier M, De Troyer A, Sampson M, et al. Aminophylline improves diaphragmatic contractility. N Engl J Med 1981;305:249–252.
200. Sigrist S, Thomas D, Howell S, et al. The effect of aminophylline on inspiratory muscle contractility. Am Rev Respir Dis 1982;126:46–50.
201. Wittmann TA, Kelsen SG. The effect of caffeine on diaphragmatic muscle force in normal hamsters. Am Rev Respir Dis 1982;126:499–504.
202. Howell S, Roussos C. Isoproterenol and aminophylline improve contractility of fatigued canine diaphragm. Am Rev Respir Dis 1984;129:118–124.
203. Aubier M, Murciano D, Viires N, et al. Increased ventilation caused by improved diaphragmatic efficiency during aminophylline infusion. Am Rev Respir Dis 1983;127:148–154.
204. Aubier M, Murciano D, Viires N, et al. Diaphragmatic contractility enhanced by aminophylline: role of extracellular calcium. J Appl Physiol 1983;54:460–464.
205. Isaacson A, Sandow A. Quinine and caffeine effects on Ca movements in frog sartorius muscle. J Gen Physiol 1967;50:2109–2128.
206. Katz AM, Repke DI, Hasselbach W. Dependence of ionophore- and caffeine-induced calcium release from sarcoplasmic reticulum vesicles on external and internal calcium ion concentrations. J Biol Chem 1977;252:1938–1949.
207. Nassar-Gentina V, Passonneau JV, Vergara JL, et al. Metabolic correlates of fatigue and of recovery from fatigue in single frog muscle fibers. J Gen Physiol 1978;72:593–606.
208. Quimbly CW, Aviado DM, Schmidt CF. The effects of aminophylline and other xanthines on the pulmonary circulation. J Pharmacol Exp Ther 1958;122:396–405.
209. Murphy GW, Schreiner BF Jr, Yu PN. Effects of aminophylline on the pulmonary circulation and left ventricular performance in patients with valvular heart disease. Circulation 1968;37:361–369.
210. Hales CA, Kazemi H. Hypoxic vascular response of the lung: effect of aminophylline and epinephrine. Am Rev Respir Dis 1974;110:126–132.
211. Blinks JR, Olson CB, Jewell BR, et al. Influence of caffeine and other methylxanthines on mechanical properties of isolated mammalian heart muscle. Evidence for a dual mechanism of action. Circ Res 1972;30:367–392.
212. Berthiaume Y, Staub NC, Matthay MA. Beta-adrenergic agonists increase lung liquid clearance in anesthetized sheep. J Clin Invest 1987;79:335–343.
213. Jayr C, Garat C, Meignan M, et al. Alveolar liquid and protein clearance in anesthetized ventilated rats. J Appl Physiol 1994;76:2636–2642.
214. Mathewson HS. Anticholinergic aerosols. Respir Care 1983;28:467–475.
215. Ziment I, Au JP. Respiratory pharmacology. Anticholinergic agents. Clin Chest Med 1986;7:355–366.
216. Motley HL, Werko L, Cournand A, et al. Observations on the clinical use of intermittent positive pressure. J Aviation Med 1947;18:417–435.

217. Cournand A, Motley HL, Werko L, et al. Physiological studies of intermittent positive pressure breathing on cardiac output in man. Am J Physiol 1948;152: 162–174.
218. Lauson HD, Bloomfield RA, Cournand A. Influence of the respiration on the circulation in man. Am J Med 1946;1:315–336.
219. Fewell JE, Abendschein DR, Carlson CJ, et al. Continuous positive-pressure ventilation decreases right and left ventricular end-diastolic volumes in the dog. Circ Res 1980;46:125–132.
220. Fewell JE, Abendschein DR, Carlson CJ, et al. Mechanism of decreased right and left ventricular end-diastolic volumes during continuous positive-pressure ventilation in dogs. Circ Res 1980;47:467–472.
221. Rankin JS, Olsen CO, Arentzen CE, et al. The effects of airway pressure on cardiac function in intact dogs and man. Circulation 1982;66:108–120.
222. Johnston WE, Vinten-Johansen J, Santamore WP, et al. Mechanism of reduced cardiac output during positive end-expiratory pressure in the dog. Am Rev Respir Dis 1989;140:1257–1264.
223. Buda AJ, Pinsky MR, Ingels NB Jr, et al. Effect of intrathoracic pressure on left ventricular performance. N Engl J Med 1979;301:453–459.
224. Jardin F, Farcot JC, Boisante L, et al. Influence of positive end-expiratory pressure on left ventricular performance. N Engl J Med 1981;304:387–392.
225. Grace MP, Greenbaum DM. Cardiac performance in response to PEEP in patients with cardiac dysfunction. Crit Care Med 1982;10:358–360.
226. Bradley TD, Holloway RM, McLaughlin PR, et al. Cardiac output response to continuous positive airway pressure in congestive heart failure. Am Rev Respir Dis 1992;145:377–382.
227. Genovese J, Moskowitz M, Tarasiuk A, et al. Effects of continuous positive airway pressure on cardiac output in normal and hypervolemic unanesthetized pigs. Am J Respir Crit Care Med 1994;150:752–758.
228. Emerson H. Artificial respiration in the treatment of edema of the lungs. Arch Intern Med 1909;3:368–371.
229. Barringer TB. Report of a case of Stokes-Adams Disease. Arch Intern Med 1909;186–189.
230. Golla FL, Symes WL. Reversible action of adrenalin and kindred drugs on the bronchioles. J Pharmacol Exp Ther 1913;5:87–103.
231. Loeb L. Mechanism in the development of pulmonary edema. Proc Soc Exp Biol Med 1928;25:321–327.
232. Cook CD, Mead J, Schreiner GL, et al. Pulmonary mechanics during induced pulmonary edema in anesthetized dogs. J Appl Physiol 1959;14:177–186.
233. Baratz DM, Westbrook PR, Shah PK, et al. Effect of nasal continuous positive airway pressure on cardiac output and oxygen delivery in patients with congestive heart failure. Chest 1992;102:1397–1401.
234. Scharf SM, Bianco JA, Tow DE, et al. The effects of large negative intrathoracic pressure on left ventricular function in patients with coronary artery disease. Circulation 1981;63:871–875.
235. Biddle TL, Khanna PK, Yu PN, et al. Lung water in patients with acute myocardial infarction. Circulation 1974;49:115–123.

Chapter 5

Pulmonary Vascular Disease and Pulmonary Hypertension:
Cardiothoracic Interactions and the Role of the Right Ventricle

David B. Badesch, M.D.

Pulmonary blood flow and cardiac performance are impacted upon by variations in intrathoracic pressure, and these interactions can be very important clinically.[1] The effects of intrathoracic pressure on left ventricular pre- and after-load are well described. This knowledge is being increasingly applied clinically in the care of patients with compromised left venticular function and volume overload.

In contrast, the performance of the right ventricle under stress is under studied, and its clinical importance under appreciated. To the clinician caring for patients with pulmonary hypertension, the importance of the relationship between pulmonary blood flow and cardiac performance is obvious. The major determinants of survival in patients with severe pulmonary hypertension relate to right ventricular performance, including cardiac output, right atrial pressure, and the pulmonary artery pressure itself.[2] In addition, it is clear that medical therapy may increase cardiac output while having minimal impact on the level of pulmonary arterial pressure elevation, and yet have a dramatic effect on the patient's functional status.

From: Cosentino AM, Martin RJ (eds.): Cardiothoracic Interrelationships in Clinical Practice. © Futura Publishing Co., Inc., Armonk, NY, 1997.

Supported by NIH Clinical Investigator Award HL 02408-04, NIH Vascular Center Award HL02825-01A1, the Pulmonary Hypertension Center at the University of Colorado, Clinical Research Center PHS RG5M01RR00051, and the Burroughs Wellcome Co.

Effects of Intrapleural Pressure on Left Ventricular Performance

General

When evaluating the determinants of pulmonary blood flow, it must be recognized that the lung circulation cannot be considered in isolation from its surroundings, including the lung parenchyma, the pleural space, and other intrathoracic structures. Permutt et al.[3–5] have eloquently described the complex interplay between the usually collapsible vessels of the lung and the pressures within the surounding tissues in their vascular waterfall paradigm.

High Levels of Peep and Auto-Peep Impair Right Ventricular Filling

The hemodynamic effects of postive end-expiratory pressure (PEEP) and auto-PEEP are frequently encountered in the intensive care unit. Increased intrathoracic/intrapleural pressures, whether caused by the extrinsic application of PEEP, by air-trapping/breath-stacking and the development of auto-PEEP,[6] or by tension pneumothorax, can impair right ventricular filling, leading to reduced cardiac output and systemic hypotension. Intravascular volume depletion potentially exacerbates the hemodynamic effects of elevated intrathoracic pressures. Treatment includes reduction of intrathoracic pressures and intravascular volume expansion. Reduction of intrathoracic pressures may be accomplished by the use of bronchodilators to relieve bronchoconstriction, increasing expiratory time by increasing the inspiratory flow rate or decreasing the respiratory rate, and perhaps by the application of extrinsic peep.

In severe congestive heart failure, positive pressure ventilation, with increased intrapleural pressures, might be of benefit due to reduced work of breathing, improved oxygenation with decreased right to left shunting (Qs/Qt), reduction of venous return,[7] and decreased left ventricular afterload (see below).

Increased Intrapleural Pressure Can Reduce Left Ventricular Afterload

Increased intrapleural pressure may improve left ventricular performance.[8,9] Furthermore, weaning from positive pressure mechanical ventilation can lead to the development of acute left ventricular dysfunction[10] and pulmonary edema. It is now well known that discontinuation of positive pressure ventilation in the pressence of intravascular volume overload and/or impaired left ventricular function can lead to the development of pulmonary edema, and consequently result in a failure to wean from the mechanical ventilator. These clinical observations are thought to be due to reduction of both pre- and after-load on the left ventricle by postive intrathoracic pressure.

Negative Intrapleural Pressure Can Increase Left Ventricular Afterload

Negative intrathoracic pressure affects left ventricular function by increasing left ventricular transmural pressures and thus afterload.[11] This may have important clinical implications. Pulmonary edema may develop in patients with negative intrathoracic pressures during acute exacerbations of asthma.[12,13] Furthermore, some investigators have proposed that chronic bronchitis and emphysema can lead to left ventricular hypertrophy and subsequent congestive heart failure.[14–16]

Cardiovascular Mechanisms of Altered Pulmonary Blood Flow

Left-Sided Valvular Heart Disease

Mitral stenosis and mitral regurgitation can lead to impairment of pulmonary blood flow and the development of pulmonary hypertension. There may be three mechanisms by which these left-sided valvular lesions lead to pulmonary hypertension: (1) a "passive" increase in pulmonary vascular resistance due to the increase in left-sided filling pressures; (2) an "active" component of pulmonary vasoconstriction; and (3) structural remodeling of the pulmonary circulation.

Left Ventricular Dysfunction

Systolic or diastolic left ventricular dysfunction can lead to the development of pulmonary hypertension. As with left-sided valvular dysfunction, increased left-sided filling pressures can lead to increased resistance to pulmonary blood flow. Diminished left ventricular systolic contractility, as seen with ischemic heart disease and dilated cardiomyopathies, and impaired relaxation and diastolic left ventricular filling, as seen in some patients with longstanding systemic hypertension and hypertrophic cardiomyopathies, can lead to increased filling pressures, with a high left atrial pressure and increased resistance to pulmonary blood flow. Severely increased left-sided resistance to pulmonary blood flow can lead to high pulmonary intravascular hydrostatic pressures and the development of pulmonary edema as described by Starling's equation (see Chapter 2). Over time, this can lead to pulmonary hemosiderosis and associated complications. Less severe elevations in left-sided filling pressures can lead to relatively subtle elevations in pulmonary artery pressures.

Pulmonary Vascular Disease

Pulmonary vascular disease can significantly impair pulmonary blood flow, resulting in a diminished cardiac output and poor organ perfusion. Vasoconstriction, structural alterations of the pulmonary vascular wall, and vascular obstruction by pulmonary thromboemboli can all lead to increased pulmonary vascular resistance and pulmonary hypertension. Because the right side of the circulation is ordinarily a high-flow, low-resistance, and low-pressure circuit, the right ventricle is poorly adapted to situations requiring sustained output in the presence of increased pulmonary vascular resistance. Abrupt increase in pulmonary vascular resistance can precipitate acute right ventricular failure, an inability to sustain cardiac output, systemic hypotension, and death. Longer-term increases in pulmonary vascular resistance can result in some adaptation of the right ventricle, with right ventricular hypertrophy. The right ventricle is better able to remain compensated if the increase in pulmonary vascular resistance occurs slowly. This is perhaps best demonstrated in those patients with pulmonary vascular disease secondary to congenital heart disease with an intracardiac shunt (see below). Ultimately, however, the right ventricle often begins to dilate, its contractility worsens, and its output decreases.

Secondary Pulmonary Hypertension

Congenital Heart Disease: The development of pulmonary hypertension due to underlying congenital heart disease is quite often insidious. It is presumed that increased flow and pressure in the pulmonary circulation, due to left-to-right intracardiac shunting, lead to structural remodeling of the pulmonary vasculature, with narrowing of the pulmonary arterial lumen and increased pulmonary vascular resistance. If the congenital defect is recognized early, prior to the development of severe pulmonary hypertension, surgical correction may prevent progression. Unfortunately, by the time patients present with dyspnea on exertion or other symptoms, pulmonary hypertension is often severe. The patient may have developed Eisenmenger physiology, with reversal of the intracardiac shunt from left-to-right to right-to-left. At this point, it may be too late to safely undertake surgical correction of the cardiac defect without simultaneous lung transplantation. The right-to-left shunt through the defect may have some protective effect on the right ventricle, preventing severe right ventricular volume overload and dilitation. The intracardiac defect may, in this situation, be serving as a "pop-off" valve. Oxygen supplementation may lessen symptoms and perhaps even slow progression of the pulmonary hypertension by preventing hypoxic vasoconstriction. However, if hypoxemia in these patients is due to a large right-to-left shunt, it may be impossible achieve a normal oxygen saturation with supplemental oxygen, particularly during physical exertion. One report suggests that pulmonary artery thrombus may be more common in patients with an underlying intracardiac shunt and pulmonary hypertension.[17]

Collagen Vascular Disease: A variety of collagen vascular diseases, including scleroderma, the CREST syndrome, systemic lupus erythematosis, and mixed connective tissue disease (MCTD), are associated with the development of pulmonary hypertension.[18–20] Pulmonary hypertension is often encountered in patients with the CREST variant of scleroderma, and less commonly in diffuse systemic sclerosis and MCTD.[21–24] The severity of pulmonary hypertension in these disorders is variable. Early vasospasm, and/or a chronic inflammatory process may contribute to the development of increased pulmonary vascular resistance in these patients.

Thromboembolic Disease: Chronic recurrent thromboembolic disease is an important potentially treatable cause of pulmonary hypertension. Appropriate prevention of pulmonary embolism is extremely important. It is now recognized that pulmonary hypertension due to chronic recurrent thromboembolic disease is often a result of structural changes in proximal pulmonary arteries causing an increase in pulmonary vascular resistance. Pulmonary emboli that have lodged in the proximal pulmonary vasculature become organized into the pulmonary arterial wall and ultimately endotheliolize. It is now possible to surgically remove such organized thrombus from the proximal pulmonary arteries of patients with pulmonary hypertension secondary to chronic recurrent thromboembolism. The Pulmonary Thromboendarterectomy Program at the University of California, San Diego has now enrolled over 500 patients, and performs approximately two such operations per week. They report that operative and perioperative mortality have improved considerably with increasing experience, and for the 150 patients done between October 1990 and March 1992 mortality was 8.7%.[25]

Hemodynamic Uniqueness of Porto-Pulmonary Hypertension: Patients with pulmonary hypertension secondary to underlying hepatic dysfunction often have a relatively preserved cardiac output. The etiology of pulmonary hypertension in this situation has been a subject of considerable discussion. It has been speculated that cytokines of other substances produced by the bowel, which are ordinarily "filtered" or processed by the liver, bypass this route in the presence of portal hypertension, and can thereby impact the lung circulation directly. Whatever the etiology, porto-pulmonary hypertension is unique in that the cardiac output is often normal or even elevated. The pulmonary vascular resistance is therefore not as elevated as in cases of pulmonary hypertension of other etiologies with comparable pulmonary arterial pressures. Furthermore, the systemic vascular resistance is often quite low in patients with severe hepatic dysfunction. Therefore, in contrast to other forms of pulmonary hypertension where the cardiac output is often decreased, porto-pulmonary hypertension is often characterized by a preserved to increased cardiac output or a high-flow state.

Primary Pulmonary Hypertension

Definition: Primary pulmonary hypertension is an often fatal disease of unknown etiology that primarily affects young women.[26] The diagnosis is one of exclusion, with known secondary causes having been ruled out. "Unexplained" pulmonary hypertension is perhaps a more appropriate term than "primary" pulmonary hypertension. "Primary" implies a single etiology, while it is more likely that this is a group of patients with heterogenous pathogenic processes that we are unable to distinquish at this time, and which share common hemodynamic manifestations and similar pathology in the late stages. The relative roles of genetic predisposition, autoimmunity, viral infection, hormonal influences, and environmental and drug exposures are not understood.[27] Based upon the recent National Institutes of Health (NIH) Registry on Primary Pulmonary Hypertension, the median survival is thought to be approximately 2.8 years from the date of diagnosis.[2]

Predictors of Survival in Primary Pulmonary Hypertension: Data from the NIH Registry on Primary Pulmonary Hypertension demonstrated that the most important predictors of survival were indices of right ventricular function, including the cardiac output and right atrial pressure, in addition to the pulmonary arterial pressure itself.[2] Sustaining or improving cardiac output therefore becomes an important therapeutic goal. We have clinically observed that treatment that improves cardiac output results in improved exercise tolerance and functional status, even in the absence of a significant fall in pulmonary arterial pressure.

Right Heart Failure and Effects on Left Ventricular Function

Compromized Left Ventricular Filling

Mechanical Compression of the Left Ventricle by the Overdistended Right Ventricle

In patients with prolonged severe pulmonary hypertension the right ventricle is often significantly dilated. This leads to an alteration in the configuration of both ventricles. While the left ventricle is ordinarily larger than the right, this size relationship can actually be reversed in the presence of severe pulmonary hypertension (Figures 1 and 2). Enlargement of the right ventricle and flattening of the interventricular septum are two characteristic

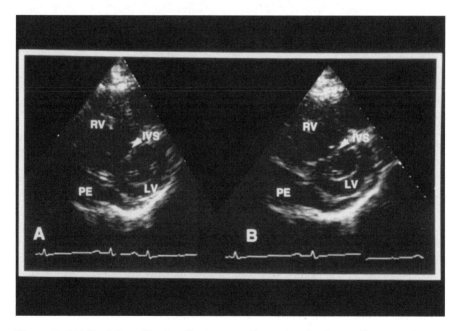

Figure 1. (A) End-diastolic view from a two-dimensional echocardiogram of a patient with severe pulmonary hypertension showing the enlarged right ventricle (RV), smaller left ventricle (LV), and flattening of the interventricular septum (IVS). A pericardial effusion (PE) is also seen. (B) End-systolic view from a two-dimensional echocardiogram of the same patient, showing the enlarged RV, smaller LV, and flattening/bowing of the IVS into the LV. The PE is again seen.

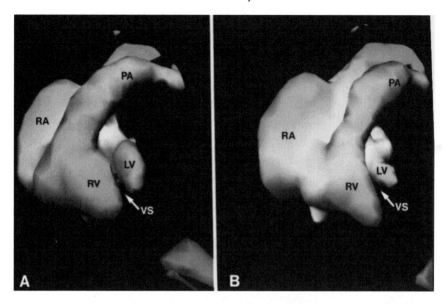

Figure 2. (A) End-diastolic view of three-dimensional MUGA scan (gated blood pool scan) of a patient with severe pulmonary hypertension, showing the massively enlarged right atrium (RA) and right ventricle (RV). The position of the interventricular septum (VS) is shown, as is the enlarged pulmonary artery (PA). (B) End-systolic view from three-dimensional MUGA scan (gated blood pool scan) of the same patient, showing the massively enlarged RV, the much smaller LV, and the position of the VS. The enlarged PA, and the massively enlarged RA are also shown.

echocardiographic findings in pateints with severe pulmonary hypertension. In some cases, the interventricular septum even bows into the left ventricular cavity, impairing diastolic filling of the left ventricle. Interventricular interdependence may interfere with the filling and output of the left ventricle.[1] The combination of impaired transit of blood across the pulmonary vascular bed, and physical impediment to left ventricular relaxation and filling may contribute to some of the syncopal episodes seen in these patients. Of note, they are also very susceptible to vaso-vagal syncope.

Optimal Filling Pressures in the Presence of Right Ventricular Failure

While patients with severe pulmonary hypertension may require higher than normal right ventricular filling pressures, there is often a point where further increases in central venous pressure lead to worsening of hemodynamics, and clinical indicators such as breathlessness, edema, and ascites. In patients with obvious volume overload due to right heart failure, it has been our practice to institute a gradual consistent diuresis until symptoms improve, or clinical evidence of impaired perfusion develops, such as a significant rise in the blood urea nitrogen or serum creatinine, or the patient demonstrates orthostatic hypotension. Abrupt reductions in right heart filling pressures should be avoided due to the risk of precipitating systemic hypotension.

Compromised Left Ventricular Contractility

Patients with severe pulmonary hypertension and right heart failure often have a flattened interventricular septum, or even bowing of the interventricular septum into the left ventricular cavity as noted above. This may lead not only to problems with left ventricular filling as discussed above, but also perhaps to decreased left ventricular contractility. This could be due to septal hypokinesis, or diminished contractility and ejection fraction related to the altered shape of the left ventricle.

Response of the Right Heart to Therapeutic Interventions

There have been several recent reviews of treatment options in patients with pulmonary hypertension.[28–30] A complete discussion of these options is beyond the scope of this chapter, but briefly they include calcium channel blockers, prostacyclin, anticoagulation (in primary pulmonary hypertension without contraindications), supplemental oxygen, diuresis when indicated, and lung or heart-lung transplantation.[31–80]

Ability of the Failing Right Ventricle to Recover Function when its Afterload is Reduced

The best example of recovery of right ventricular function comes from the transplant experience. It was previously thought that heart-lung transplantation was required for patients with severe pulmonary hypertension, due to the decompensated state of the right ventricle. However, it is now clear that the right ventricle has a remarkable ability to recover function when it is unloaded and downstream resistance to flow is decreased.[64,66,70,71,75,76,79] In addition, reparable congenital heart defects, such as ASDs and some VSDs can be closed at the time of lung transplantation, allowing the patient to keep their native heart. Keeping one's own heart is preferable if possible due to the risk of rejection of the heart and accelerated coronary atherosclerosis. In addition, some experts believe that patients receiving heart-lung transplants are at increased risk for rejection of the lungs relative to patients receiving lungs only. Finally, lung, as opposed to heart-lung, transplantation conserves precious donor organs, allowing transplantation of more patients. Heart-lung transplantation is still required in patients with pulmonary hypertension secondary to complex congenital heart defects that are not feasible to repair at the time of lung transplantation.

Pulmonary Perfusion Problems Unique to Patients Undergoing Single Lung Transplantation for Primary Pulmonary Hypertension

Patients receiving lung transplants are at risk for postoperative edema thought secondary to ischemia-reperfusion. This problem may be exacerbated in the pulmonary hypertensive patient undergoing single lung transplantation due to the fact that almost all of the patient's pulmonary blood flow will go to the new lung (due to the very high resistance to flow in the remaining native lung). This may create dramatic physiologic disturbances due to ventilation-perfusion mismatching, with the great majority of blood flow going to the new lung, and the majority of ventilation going to the the non-edematous, more compliant, native lung. Extreme cases may require independent lung ventilation through a dual-lumen endotracheal tube using two ventilators.[81] Episodes of rejection in patients receiving single-lung transplantation for pulmonary hypertension may also lead to very significant ventilation-perfusion mismatching. For these reasons double lung transplantation may be preferred for patients with pulmonary hypertension, despite being a longer, more complicated operation, likely with a slightly higher operative mortality rate. Obviously though, double-lung transplantation is less organ-conserving. Our approach has been to list younger patients with pulmonary hypertension for double lung transplants.

Acknowledgment: Figures kindly provided by Robert A. Quaife, M.D., Division of Cardiology, University of Colorado Health Sciences Center.

References

1. Butler J. The heart is not always in good hands. Chest 1990;97:453–460.
2. D'Alonzo GE, Barst RJ, Ayres SM, et al. Survival in patients with primary pulmonary hypertension. Results from a national prospective registry. Ann Intern Med 1991;115:343–349.
3. Permutt S, Riley RL. Hemodynamics of collapsible vessels with tone: The vascular waterfall. J Appl Physiol 1963;18:924–932.
4. Permutt S, Bromberger-Barnea B, Bane HN. Alveolar pressure, pulmonary venous pressure, and the vascular waterfall. Med Thorac 1962;19:239–260.
5. Permutt S, Wise RA, Sylvester JT. Interaction between the circulatory and ventilatory pumps. In: Lenfant C (ed). Lung Biology in Health and Disease, Volume 29. New York, Marcel Dekker, 1985, pp. 701–735.

6. Pepe PE, Marini JJ. Occult positive end-expiratory pressure in mechanically ventilated patients with airflow obstruction. The auto-PEEP effect. Am Rev Respir Dis 1982;126:166–170.

7. Slustky AS. Consensus conference on mechanical ventilation January 28–30, 1993 at Northbrook, Illinois, USA. Int Care Med 1994;20:64–79.

8. Suter PM, Fairley HB, Isenberg MD. Optimum end-expiratory pressure in patients with acute pulmonary failure. N Engl J Med 1975;292:284–289.

9. Pinsky MR, et al. Augmentation of cardiac function by elevation of intrathoracic pressure. J Appl Physiol 1983;54:950–955.

10. Lemaire F, et al. Acute left ventricular dysfunction during unsuccessful weaning from mechanical ventilation. Anesthesiology 1988;69:171–179.

11. Buda AJ, Pinsky MR, Ingels NB Jr, et al. Effect of intrathoracic pressure on left ventricular performance. N Engl J Med 1979;301:453–459.

12. Stalcup SA, Mellins RB. Mechanical forces producing pulmonary edema in acute asthma. N Engl J Med 1977;297:592–596.

13. Luke MJ, Mehrizi A, Forger GM Jr, et al. Chronic nasopharyngeal obstruction as a cause of cardiomegaly, *cor pulmonale,* and pulmonary edema. Pediatrics 1966;37:762–768.

14. Michelson N. Bilateral ventricular hypertrophy due to chronic pulmonary disease. Dis Chest 1960;38:435–446.

15. Fluck DC, Chandrasekar RG, Gardner RV. Left ventricular hypertrophy in chronic bronchitis. Br Heart J 1966;28:92–97.

16. Rao BS, Cohn KE, Eldridge FL. Left ventricular failure secondary to chronic pulmonary disease. Am J Med 1968;45:229–241.

17. Schamroth CL, Sareli P, Pocock WA, et al. Pulmonary arterial thrombosis in secundum atrial septal defect. Am J Cardiol 1987;60:1152–1156.

18. Salerni R, Rodnan GP, Leon DF, et al. Pulmonary hypertension in the CREST syndrome variant of progressive systemic sclerosis (scleroderma). Ann Intern Med 1977;86:394–399.

19. Kanemoto N, Gonda N, Katsu M, et al. Case report. Two cases of pulmonary hypertension with Raynoud's Phenomenon. Primary pulmonary hypertension and systemic lupus erythematosis. Jpn Heart J 1975;16:354–360.

20. Graziano FM, Friedman LC, Grossman J. Pulmonary hypertension in a patient with mixed connective tissue disease: Clinical and pathologic findings, and review of the literature. Clin Exp Rheumatol 1983;1:251–255.

21. Alpert MA, Pressly TA, Mukerji V, et al. Short- and long-term hemodynamic effects of captopril in patients with pulmonary hypertension and selected connective tissue disease. Chest 1992;102:1407–1412.

22. Ungerer R, Tashkin D, Furst D, et al. Prevalence and clinical correlates of pulmonary arterial hypertension in progressive systemic sclerosis. Am J Med 1983;75:65–74.

23. Alpert M, Goldberg S, Singsen B, et al. Cardiovascular manifestations of mixed connective tissue disease in adults. Circulation 1983;68:1182–1193.

24. Kasukawa R, Nishimaki T, Takagi T, et al. Pulmonary hypertension in connective tissue disease. Clinical analysis of sixty patients in a multi-institutional study. Clin Rheum 1990;9:56–62.

25. Jamieson SW, Auger WR, Fidulo PF, et al. Experience and results with 150 pulmonary thromboendarterectomy operations over a 29 month period. J Thorac Cardiovasc Surg 1993;106:116–127.

26. Rich S, Dantzker DR, Ayres SM, et al. Primary pulmonary hypertension. A national prospective study. Ann Intern Med 1987;107:216–223.

27. Badesch DB, Wynne KM, Bonvallet S, et al. Hypothyroidism and primary pulmonary hypertension: An autoimmune pathogenetic link? Ann Intern Med 1993;119:44–46.
28. Badesch DB, Groves BM. Current therapeutic options in severe pulmonary hypertension. Sem Resp Med 1994;15:482–489.
29. Rubin LJ, Chairman, ACCP Consensus Conference. ACCP Consensus Statement. Primary pulmonary hypertension. Chest 1993;104:236–250.
30. Rubin LJ. Primary pulmonary hypertension: Practical therapeutic recommendations. Drugs 1992;43:37–43.
31. DeFeyter PJ, Kerkkamp HJ, de Jong JP. Sustained beneficial effect of nifedipine in primary pulmonary hypertension. Am Heart J 1983;105:333–334.
32. Groves BM, Badesch DB, Turkevich D, et al. Correlation of acute prostacyclin response in primary (unexplained) pulmonary hypertension with efficacy of treatment with calcium channel blockers and survival. In: Weir K (ed). The Role of Ion Flux in Pulmonary Vascular Control. New York, Plenum Publishing Corporation, 1993.
33. Lunde P, Rasmussen K. Long-term beneficial effect of nifedipine in primary pulmonary hypertension. Am Heart J 1984;108:415–416.
34. Olivari MT, Levine TB, Weir EK, et al. Hemodynamic effects of nifedepine at rest and during exercise in primary pulmonary hypertension. Chest 1984;86:14–19.
35. Rich S, Brundage BH. High-dose calcium channel-blocking therapy for primary pulmonary hypertension: Evidence for long-term reduction in pulmonary arterial pressure and regression of right ventricular hypertrophy. Circulation 1987;76:135–141.
36. Rich S, Kaufman E, Levy PS. The effect of high doses of calcium-channel blockers on survival in primary pulmonary hypertension. N Engl J Med 1992;327:76–81.
37. Rubin LJ, Nicod P, Hillis LD, et al. Treatment of primary pulmonary hypertension with nifedipine. Ann Intern Med 1983;99:433–437.
38. Saito D, Haraoka S, Yoshida H, et al. Primary pulmonary hypertension improved by long-term oral administration of nifedipine. Am Heart J 1983;105:1041–1042.
39. Barst RJ, Rubin LJ, McGoon MD, et al. Survival in primary pulmonary hypertension with long-term continuous intravenous prostacyclin. Ann Intern Med 1994;121:409–415.
40. Christman BW, McPherson CD, Newman JH, et al. An imbalance between the excretion of thromboxane and prostacyclin metabolites in pulmonary hypertension. N Engl J Med 1992;327:70–75.
41. Hyman AL, Kadowitz PJ. Pulmonary vasodilator activity of prostacyclin in the cat. Circ Res 1979;45:404.
42. Jones DK, Higginbottam TW, Wallwork J. Treatment of primary pulmonary hypertension with intravenous epoprostenol (prostacyclin). Br Heart J 1987;57:270–278.
43. Long W, Rubin L, Barst R, et al. Randomized trial of conventional therapy alone [CT] vs. conventional therapy + continuous infusions of prostacyclin [CT + PGI$_2$] in primary pulmonary hypertension (PPH): A 12 week study. (abstract) Am Rev Respir Dis 1993;147:A538.
44. Moncada S, Gryglewski RJ, Bunting S, et al. An enzyme isolated from arteries transforms prostaglandin endoperoxides to an unstable substance that inhibits platelet aggregation. Nature 1976;263:633.

45. Moncada S, Vane JR. Arachidonic acid metabolites and the interactions between platelets and blood vessel walls. N Engl J Med 1979;300:1142.
46. Rubin LJ, Groves BM, Reeves JT, et al. Prostacyclin-induced pulmonary vasodilation in primary pulmonary hypertension. Circulation 1982;66:334–338.
47. Rubin LJ, Mendoza J, Hood M, et al. Treatment of primary pulmonary hypertension with continuous intravenous prostacyclin (epoprostenol). Results of a randomized trial. Ann Intern Med 1990;112:485–491.
48. Fuster V, et al. Primary pulmonary hypertension: Natural history and importance of thrombosis. Circulation 1984;70:580–587.
49. Bohlman RM, Shumway SJ, Estrin JA, et al. Lung and heart-lung transplantation. Evolution and new applications. Ann Surg 1991;214:456–468.
50. Chapelier A, Vouhe P, Macchiarini P, et al. Comparative outcome of heart-lung and lung transplantation for pulmonary hypertension. J Thorac Cardiovasc Surg 1993;106:299–307.
51. Glanville AR, Baldwin JC, Hunt SA, et al. Long-term cardiopulmonary function after human heart-lung transplantation. Aust N Z J Med 1990;20:208–214.
52. Griffith BP, Hardesty RL, Armitage JM, et al. A decade of lung transplantation. Ann Surg 1993;218:310–318.
53. Higgenbottam TW, Spiegelhalter D, Scott JP, et al. Prostacyclin (epoprostenol) and heart-lung transplantation as treatments for severe pulmonary hypertension. Br Heart J 1993;70:366–370.
54. Jamieson SW, Stinson EB, Oyer PE, et al. Heart-lung transplantation for irreversible pulmonary hypertension. Ann Thorac Surg 1984;38:554–562.
55. Kramer MR, Marshall SE, Tiroke A, et al. Clinical significance of hyperbilirubinemia in patients with pulmonary hypertension undergoing heart-lung transplantation. J Heart Lung Transplant 1991;10:317–321.
56. McCarthy PM, Kirby TJ, White RD, et al. Lung and heart-lung transplantation: State of the art. Cleve Clin J Med 1992;59:307–316.
57. Reitz BA, Wallwork JL, Hunt SA, et al. Heart-lung transplantation: Successful therapy for patients with pulmonary vascular disease. N Engl J Med 1982;306: 557–564.
58. Rhenman B, Rhenman MJ, Icenogle TB, et al. Heart-lung transplantation: The initial Arizona experience. J Thorac Cardiovasc Surg 1989;98:922–927.
59. Theodore J, Morris AJ, Burke CM, et al. Cardiopulmonary function at maximum tolerable constant work rate exercise following human heart-lung transplantation. Chest 1987;92:433–439.
60. UNOS (United Network for Organ Sharing) Organ Procurement and Transplantation Network Data and UNOS Scientific Registry. UNOS Update. Volume 9, Issue 5, May 1993. Richmond, Virginia.
61. Bolman RM III, Shumway SJ, Estrin JA, et al. Lung and heart-lung transplantation. Evolution and new applications. Ann Surg 1991;214:456–468.
62. Calhoon JH, Grover FL, Gibbons WJ, et al. Single lung transplantation. Alternative indications and technique. J Thorac Cardiovasc Surg 1991;101:816–824.
63. de Hoyos AL, Patterson GA, Maurer JR, et al. Pulmonary transplantation. Early and late results. The Toronto Lung Transplant Group. J Thorac Cardiovasc Surg 1992;103:295–306.
64. Fremmes SE, Patterson GA, Williams WG, et al. Single lung transplantation and closure of patent ductus arteriosus for Eisenmenger's syndrome. Toronto Lung Transplant Group. J Thorac Cardiovasc Surg 1990;100:1–5.
65. Frist WH, Loyd JE, Merrill WH, et al. Single lung transplantation: A temporal look at rejection, infection, and survival. Am Surg 1994;60:94–102.

66. Globits S, Burghuber OC, Koller J, et al. Effect of lung transplantation on right and left ventricular volumes and function measured by magnetic resonance imaging. Am J Respir Crit Care Med 1994;149:1000–1004.
67. Hayden AM, Robert RC, Kriett JM, et al. Primary diagnosis predicts prognosis of lung transplant candidates. Transplantation 1993;55:1048–1050.
68. Haydock DA, Trulock EP, Kaiser LR, et al. Lung transplantation. Analysis of thirty-six consecutive procedures performed over a twelve-month period. The Washington University Lung Transplant Group. J Thorac Cardiovasc Surg 1992;103:329–340.
69. Ichiba S, Okabe K, Date H, et al. Experimental study on veno-venous extracorporeal membrane oxygenation for respiratory failure after lung transplantation. Acta Med Okayama 1992;46:213–221.
70. Kramer MR, Valantine HA, Marshall SE, et al. Recovery of the right ventricle after single-lung transplantation in pulmonary hypertension. Am J Cardiol 1994; 73:494–500.
71. Levine SM, Gibbons WJ, Bryan CL, et al. Single lung transplantation for primary pulmonary hypertension. Chest 1990;98:1107–1115.
72. Levine SM, Jenkinson SG, Bryan CL, et al. Ventilation-perfusion inequalities during graft rejection in patients undergoing single lung transplantation for primary pulmonary hypertension. Chest 1992;101:401–405.
73. Lupinetti FM, Bolling SF, Bove EL, et al. Selective lung or heart-lung transplantation for pulmonary hypertension associated with congenital cardiac anomalies. Ann Thorac Surg 1994;57:1545–1548.
74. Nootens M, Freels S, Kaufman E, et al. Timing of single lung transplantation for primary pulmonary hypertension. J Heart Lung Transplant 1994;13:276–281.
75. Pasque MK, Trulock EP, Kaiser LR, et al. Single-lung transplantation for pulmonary hypertension. Three-month hemodynamic follow-up. Circulation 1991; 84:2275–2279.
76. Ritchie M, Waggoner AD, Davila-Roman VG, et al. Echocardiographic characterization of the improvement in right ventricular function in patients with severe pulmonary hypertension after single-lung transplantation. J Am Coll Cardiol 1993;22:1170–1174.
77. Sikela ME, Noon GP, Holland VA, et al. Differential perfusion: Potential complication of femoral-femoral bypass during single lung transplantation. Heart Lung Transplant 1991;10:322–324.
78. Patterson GA, Lappas DG. Predictors, frequency, and indications for cardiopulmonary bypass during lung transplantation in adults. Ann Thorac Surg 1994;57:1248–1251.
79. Cooper JD, Patterson GA, Trulock EP. Results of single and bilateral lung transplantation in 131 consecutive recipients. Washington University Lung Transplant Group. J Thorac Cardiovasc Surg 1994;107:460–470.
80. Kaiser LR, Cooper JD. The current status of lung transplantation. Adv Surg 1992;25:259–307.
81. Badesch DB, Zamora M, Jones S, et al. Independent ventilation and extracorporeal membrane oxygenation (ECMO) for severe unilateral pulmonary edema following single lung transplantation for primary (unexplained) pulmonary hypertension. Chest (In Press).

Chapter 6

Pulmonary Hypertension in Status Asthmaticus

Thomas Corbridge, M.D., Jesse B. Hall, M.D.

Asthma is a disease characterized by wheezing, dyspnea, and cough resulting from airway inflammation, airway hyperreactivity, and variable degrees of reversible airflow obstruction.[1,2] Asthma afflicts up to 10 million people in the United States, and the number of cases is on the rise.[2] Fortunately, most patients do not have debilitating disease and symptoms are easily controlled with education and a limited number of medications. But in others, this disease paints a much more malignant picture of daily breathlessness and severe functional impairment—much like patients with emphysema and fixed airflow limitation.

All patients with asthma are at risk of developing a severe asthma attack—a disorder called "status asthmaticus" (SA). Attacks may be sudden when smooth muscle mediated bronchospasm acutely increases airflow obstruction, or slowly progressive when there is worsening airway wall inflammation. No matter the tempo, this life-threatening disorder results in multiple derangements in pulmonary function. Well known among these changes are airflow obstruction, lung hyperinflation, increased work of breathing, and gas exchange abnormalities.

With the exception of pulsus paradoxus (PP), cardiovascular complications of acute asthma have received much less attention. The presence of sinus tachycardia and various atrial, ventricular, and combined rhythm disturbances have been described,[3,4] and there are concerns that acute asthma may lead to myocardial oxygen supply/demand imbalance and myocardial

From: Cosentino AM, Martin RJ (eds.): Cardiothoracic Interrelationships in Clinical Practice. © Futura Publishing Co., Inc., Armonk, NY, 1997.

ischemia.[5] Less well appreciated is that patients with SA can develop pulmonary hypertension.

Patients with SA may have exam findings of pulmonary hypertension including accentuation of the pulmonic component of the second heart sound, jugular venous distention, and occasionally a right-sided third heart sound. In addition, electrocardiographic findings of right axis deviation, clockwise rotation, and right ventricular hypertrophy have been described that resolve within hours of successful treatment.[6] There appears to be more behind these electrocardiographic changes than simply the vertical position of the heart in the hyperinflated chest.

The incidence and clinical importance of pulmonary hypertension in SA are not known. Moreover, etiologic factors contributing to the development of pulmonary hypertension have not been extensively studied and are therefore not entirely understood. Although there may be a dominant mechanism, it is likely that pulmonary hypertension in SA is the result of the interaction of several different mechanisms.

Among these mechanisms are the mechanical effects of airflow obstruction, and its consequence, lung hyperinflation, on pulmonary vascular resistance. Other contributing factors may be restriction of cardiac movement within the cardiac fossa, an increase in cardiac output in the setting of functional vascular obstruction, alterations in arterial blood gases, and the release of various mediators of pulmonary vasomotor tone.

In this chapter, each of these possible etiologic factors is reviewed in turn. We finish by reviewing pharmacologic and ventilatory strategies used in the treatment of SA with regard to their possible effects on the severity of pulmonary hypertension, and discuss whether, or not, treatment other than that aimed at reversal of airflow obstruction is indicated.

Airflow Obstruction

Patients with asthma invariably demonstrate physiologic evidence of expiratory airflow obstruction, which worsens over hours to days during acute attacks. Often, a simple physical examination maneuver is enough to establish airflow obstruction and delayed lung emptying—such as timing a patient's forced expiration from total lung capacity (TLC) during chest auscultation. Better, is the use of a spirometer or peak expiratory flow rate meter to assess the degree of airflow obstruction. Alternately, airway resistance or its inverse, airway conductance, can be measured directly in a body plethysmograph.

Airflow obstruction in asthma is influenced by a number of factors including smooth muscle mediated bronchoconstriction, smooth muscle hypertrophy, intraluminal mucus, and airway edema, all of which appear to be initiated by airway wall inflammation. A number of cells including eosinophils, mast cells, macrophages, neutrophils, and epithelial cells are involved in this inflammatory process.

In patients who die with SA, postmortem examination of the lungs often demonstrates extensive mucus plugging of large and small airways along with diffuse shedding of the epithelial lining and a denuded basement membrane. The pathology of sudden asphyxic asthma may be quite different from asthma that progresses slowly over hours to days.[7] Recent studies have demonstrated that patients dying suddenly in SA have diminished eosinophils and increased neutrophils in the airway submucosa,[8] and less intraluminal mucus,[9] compared to patients with slower onset disease.

Lung Hyperinflation

Airflow obstruction prolongs the time constant of the respiratory system, delays lung emptying, and causes lung hyperinflation. A time constant is the time it takes a viscoelastic object to reach a new point of equilibrium after it is distorted. For the lung, the time constant is defined as the product of resistance and compliance. In SA, increased airway resistance prolongs the time constant—even though this effect is partially attenuated by patients breathing at large lung volumes and on the flat (or less compliant) portion of the pressure-volume curve (Figure 1). In asthma, it takes longer during exhalation to reach resting lung volume— the amount of air in the lung at the end of a tidal breath, or functional residual capacity (FRC).

When inspiration occurs before there is complete emptying of alveolar gas, dynamic lung hyperinflation occurs and FRC increases. Alveolar gas is "trapped" in areas with long time constants (i.e., areas supplied by narrowed airways) and alveolar pressure remains positive at the end of expiration. This phenomenon is referred to as auto-positive end-expiratory pressure, or auto-PEEP. Short exhalation times, such as occur with hyperventilation, further aggravate this dynamic lung hyperinflation. With successful treatment of the acute asthma attack, airflow obstruction is diminished, lung emptying is more complete, and lung volumes decrease.

Changes in static mechanics also influence FRC in asthma. FRC is a point of equilibrium determined by the outward recoil of the chest wall and the inward elastic recoil of the lung. In asthma with long standing lung hyperinflation, there may be loss of lung elastic recoil (which increases FRC). Also, persistent inspiratory muscle activity during expiration may increase outward recoil of the chest further elevating FRC.

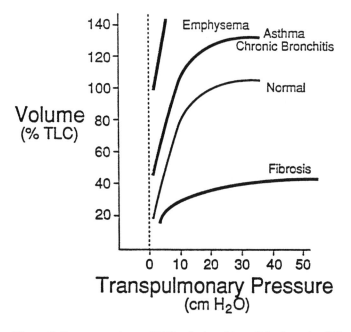

Figure 1. Pressure-volume (P-V) relationships of the lung in different lung diseases. In normal subjects, TLC is established when the P-V curve of the lung plateaus. In asthma, the P-V curve is classically shifted upward and to the left, with a normal slope, and TLC is elevated. In patients with emphysema, the P-V curve of the lung is shifted upward and to the left with an increased slope indicating loss of lung elastic recoil. Conversely in pulmonary fibrosis, the P-V curve is shifted downward and to the right with a decreased slope indicating increased elastic recoil (decreased lung compliance). Note that in normal subjects and in patients with asthma, lung compliance (i.e., the slope of P-V curve), decreases at high lung volumes. (From Corbridge T, Irvin CG. Pathophysiology of chronic obstructive pulmonary disease with emphasis on physiologic and pathologic correlations. In: Casaburi R, Petty T (eds). Principles and Practice of Pulmonary Rehabilitation. Philadelphia, PA, W. B. Saunders Co., 1993, p. 19,[57] with permission).

TLC is the volume of gas present after a full inflation. In health, TLC is determined by the ability to inspire (requiring adequate strength and effort) and by the pressure-volume characteristics of the lung parenchyma. When a full inflation occurs, TLC is established when the pressure-volume curve of the lung plateaus. In asthma, the pressure-volume curve is classically shifted upward and to the left, with a normal slope, and TLC is elevated (Figure 1).

Residual volume (RV) is the volume of gas in the lungs at the end of a maximal exhalation. It is determined by a patient's ability to exhale completely (again requiring adequate strength and effort) and by airway closure.

In young, healthy persons, RV may be limited by pain, but in older subjects RV is more often determined by airway closure. In asthma, RV is elevated because airway narrowing prevents complete emptying of alveolar gas.

Benefits of Lung Hyperinflation

Lung volume is an important determinant of lung function—particularly maximal expiratory airflow. There are two main explanations for this relationship. First, as lung volume increases, lung elastic recoil increases and lung compliance decreases (pressure-volume relationship). As stated above, decreased lung compliance shortens the time constant, increases expiratory airflow, and thereby aids in the exhalation of gas during periods of worsening lung hyperinflation. Second, as lung volume increases, airways expand because of the tethering effect of the surrounding lung parenchyma. This maintains airway patency, lowers airway resistance, and protects expiratory airflow.

Disadvantages of Lung Hyperinflation

Disadvantages of lung hyperinflation include a decrease in the pressure-generating ability of the diaphragm, an increase pulmonary vascular resistance (PVR), possible adverse effects on the cardiac fossa, and an increase in work of breathing requiring patients to generate wide swings in pleural pressure (Ppl) to maintain adequate flow of air.

Effects on Diaphragm Function

Two common explanations have been put forth to explain the effects of lung hyperinflation on inspiratory diaphragm function. First, lung hyperinflation flattens (and thereby increases the radius of curvature) of the diaphragm. By Laplace's equation, this conformational change results in less pressure-generating ability. Second, hyperinflation reduces precontractile muscle length, which by the known relationship between length and tension in skeletal muscle, decreases muscle tension developed during contraction.

Lung Inflation and Pulmonary Vascular Resistance

To understand how lung hyperinflation increases PVR, we must explain the difference between the two main types of intrapulmonary blood vessels, the alveolar and extra-alveolar vessels. These two vessel types are distinguished from each other by their location in the lung and by the opposite effects of lung expansion and contraction to expand and compress these vessels.[10] The smaller alveolar vessels abut airspaces where they are involved in gas exchange and where they are influenced by changes in alveolar pressure (P_A). When lung volume increases either by a spontaneous negative pressure breath or by positive pressure ventilation, P_A increases relative to Ppl, increasing transpulmonary pressure ($Ptm=P_A$-Ppl). Lung inflation compresses and narrows alveolar vessels and increases resistance to the flow of blood through them.[11]

Extra-alveolar vessels are larger intrapulmonary vessels that do not border airspaces. The pressure surrounding these vessels is approximated by Ppl. As the lung expands, there is an increase in the capacitance of the peribronchovascular interstitium where extra-alveolar vessels lie as the alveolar septa pull in radial fashion on the connective tissue sheath surrounding these vessels. Contrary to effects on alveolar vessels, lung inflation expands extra-alveolar vessels and decreases the resistance to flow through them.

Thus as lung volume increases, alveolar vessels are compressed and extra-alveolar vessels are distended, increasing and decreasing resistance to pulmonary blood flow through each vessel type, respectively. Conversely, low lung volumes may distort extra-alveolar vessels and increase resistance to blood flow through them. Total PVR is minimized around resting lung volume (FRC)[12,13] such that increases in lung volume above FRC increase PVR and decreases in lung volume below FRC increase PVR (Figure 2). A biphasic relationship thereby exists between lung inflation and PVR.[14–16] By way of example, in acute lung injury states, lung edema and atelectasis combine to decrease lung volume and increase PVR. Ventilator applied positive end-expiratory pressure (PEEP) redistributes alveolar edema into the surrounding interstitium and recruits lung volume. As lung volume increases, PVR decreases until higher levels of applied PEEP increase PVR through lung hyperinflation.[17] Recruitment of alveoli in acute lung injury states also improves alveolar oxygenation to decrease hypoxic pulmonary vasoconstriction and its contribution to higher PVR (see below).

Harris and colleagues[18] studied the effects of hyperventilation on PVR in normal patients and in patients with chronic bronchitis. PVR (dynes sec cm^{-5}) was calculated by dividing the pressure change across the pulmonary circulation (mean Ppa-pulmonary capillary wedge pressure or Pw) (mmHg) by pulmonary blood flow (L/min). Among normal subjects, hyperventilation had no significant effect on Ppa, Pw, or PVR. In contrast, hyperventilation in patients with chronic bronchitis caused a consistent increase in Pw (from 9 mmHg to 18 mmHg) and an even greater increase in Ppa (from 28 mmHg to 43 mmHg) thus increasing the pressure gradient across the pulmonary circulation. Pulmonary blood flow did not change. Thus, on average, there was an increase in PVR (from 457 dynes sec cm^{-5} to 607 dynes sec cm^{-5}). The authors concluded that in patients with chronic bronchitis

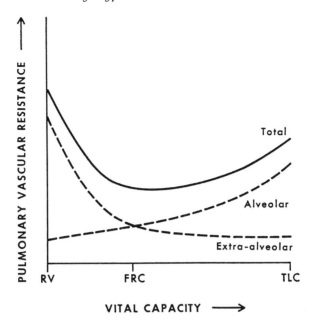

Figure 2. Total pulmonary vascular resistance (and the contributions of alveolar and extra-alveolar vessels to the total) as a function of lung volume. As lung volume increases from residual volume (RV), resistance to flow in extra-alveolar vessels decreases, whereas resistance in alveolar vessels increases. Total pulmonary vascular resistance is at its lowest around at functional residual capacity (FRC). (From Murray JF. Circulation. In: Murray JF (ed). The Normal Lung. The Basis for Diagnosis and Treatment of Pulmonary Disease. Philadelphia, PA, W. B. Saunders Co., 1976, p.131, with permission).

and increased expiratory airway resistance, hyperventilation resulted in lung hyperinflation, increased P_A, and compression of the resistance (alveolar) vessels in the lung. In normal subjects, however, low airways resistance allowed for complete lung emptying despite hyperventilation and protected against lung hyperinflation. In the same study, mean alveolar pressure was increased in normal subjects by increasing airway pressure at the mouth. By encircling the chest wall with a rubber strain gauge, subjects voluntarily kept FRC within the normal range. Under these conditions, increasing P_A increased the slope of the relationship between lung blood flow and the pressure gradient across the pulmonary circulation, again indicating an increase in PVR.

In SA, it is likely that lung hyperinflation compresses alveolar vessels and increases PVR. This effect may be unequal because lung units are variably hyperinflated. It is likely that alveolar vessels have a wide range of resistances related to their adjacent P_A and that vascular resistance is highest in lung units with the most trapped air. Increased PVR from lung hyperinflation may be a leading factor in increasing right ventricular afterload and Ppa in patients with SA.[19,20]

Effects on the Cardiac Fossa

Lung hyperinflation (and decreased lung compliance) may restrict movement of the walls of the cardiac fossa.[21] The hyperinflated lung is more difficult to deform,[22] and may interfere with cardiac movement. Theoretically, this restriction to movement may increase afterload and decrease compliance of both ventricles. Over time, the added load may contribute to the development of right heart failure in patients with long standing, severe lung hyperinflation, such as in chronic obstructive pulmonary disease (COPD). This mechanism may also help explain the appearance of left ventricular hypertrophy in some of these patients as well.[21] Effects of acute lung hyperinflation (such as occurs in SA) on cardiac movement are not well understood.

Work of Breathing

Airflow obstruction and lung hyperinflation increase work of breathing by increasing airway resistance and decreasing lung compliance, respectively. In asthma, work of breathing may be 5 to 10 times normal. During inspiration, patients must generate significant muscle force (as measured by the drop in Ppl) to overcome the effects of auto-PEEP and increased inspiratory airway resistance. Since auto-PEEP is positive alveolar pressure at the initiation of an inspiratory effort, Ppl must drop below the level of auto-PEEP before a pressure gradient is created between mouth and alveolus sufficient for airflow to occur. During expiration, Ppl must be sufficiently great to overcome expiratory airway resistance (which increases as the lung deflates). When muscle force is not adequate (through mechanical effects of hyperinflation and/or fatigue) to overcome flow-resistive and elastic loads, airflow is not maintained, and respiratory failure ensues.

In SA, Ppl often decreases to -20 to -40 cmH$_2$O during inspiration and increases to 7 to 10 cmH$_2$O during expiration (compared to approximately -8 cmH$_2$O during inspiration and -4 cmH$_2$O during expiration in the normal quiet state).[23–26] The reason that the magnitude of change in Ppl is greater during inspiration than expiration (despite lower airway resistance during inspiration) is, in part, that patients must overcome the effects of auto-PEEP. Also, during expiration, lung elastic pressure (Pel) adds to Ppl to generate alveolar pressure (Palv) (Palv = Ppl + Pel), which is the driving pressure for expiratory airflow.

Effects of Changes in Pleural Pressures

Both the pulmonary artery and left atrium are surrounded by Ppl. Accordingly, changes in Ppl that occur with respiration affect both Ppa and Pla (as estimated by Pw). During a normal spontaneous inspiration, Ppl drops and lowers both Ppa and Pla—although the driving pressure across the pulmonary system (Ppa-Pla) stays the same. Conversely, during a positive pressure breath, Ppl increases and raises both Ppa and Pla. Ventilator applied PEEP raises Ppa and Pla throughout the respiratory cycle by increasing Ppl.

As with ventilator applied PEEP, auto-PEEP increases intraluminal vascular pressures by increasing Ppl, although effects may be less uniform because of asymmetric air trapping. The magnitude with which auto-PEEP affects Ppl in asthma is not known. For ventilator applied PEEP in the setting of relaxed respiratory muscles, the change in Ppl in response to PEEP depends on the compliance of both the lung (C_L) and chest wall (C_W). The formula deltaPpl = PEEP X $C_L/(C_L + C_W)$ predicts that in normal lungs half of the applied PEEP is transmitted to the pleural space, because C_L and C_W are roughly equal in normal subjects in the tidal volume range.[27] This formula also demonstrates that less PEEP is transmitted to the pleural space when lungs are stiff as in pulmonary edema or when there is significant lung hyperinflation. In patients with obstructive diseases who are not in exacerbation, however, vascular effects of applied PEEP or auto-PEEP may be accentuated by the loss of lung elasticity and increased lung compliance characteristic of the stable state.

The Concept of Transmural Pressure

Effects of respiration on vascular pressures are readily seen on the pulmonary artery catheter tracing. It is important to point out, however, that pressures measured by the pulmonary artery catheter are intraluminal—not transmural—pressures. That is, pulmonary artery catheter derived pressures are referenced to atmospheric pressure—not to Ppl. The more interesting pressure, of course, is transmural pressure because it reflects the true distending or filling pressure of the vessel. Transmural pressure is the difference in pressure between intraluminal vascular pressure (e.g., Ppa) and the pressure outside of the vessel—usually estimated by Ppl. During quiet breathing, transmural pressure is close to intraluminal pressure because Ppl is small. But transmural pressure can vary greatly from intraluminal pressure when states like asthma significantly change Ppl.

Intraluminal and transmural pressures can track in opposite directions during the respiratory cycle. By way of example, Gunstone demonstrated that intraluminal right heart or pulmonary artery pressures fall in SA because of large drops in Ppl (see below).[28] However, in the face of lower Ppa, patients developed electrocardiographic signs of right heart strain. This finding is explained by an increase in transmural Ppa (because Ppl dropped more than Ppa) and an increase in right ventricular afterload. Similarly, in their study of the mechanism of PP in SA, Jardin and coworkers,[25] demonstrated a fall in mean systolic and diastolic Ppa during inspiration from 37.0 to 11.1 mmHg, and 20.4 to −2.8 mmHg, respectively. But because mean Ppl (estimated by esophageal balloon) was 7.6 mmHg during expiration and −24.4 mmHg during inspiration, pulmonary artery transmural systolic pressure increased from 29.4 mmHg (37.0 −7.6 mmHg) during expiration to 35.5 mmHg during inspiration. Likewise, pulmonary artery transmural diastolic pressure increased from 12.8 mmHg during expiration to 21.6 mmHg during inspiration.

During their study of acute asthma exacerbation triggered by ragweed aerosol, Permut and colleagues[19] found that end-inspiratory Ppl fell by an average of 20 cmH$_2$O and the Ppa relative to Ppl (transmural Ppa) increased by about the same amount (despite a drop in intraluminal Ppa). A tenable explanation for the close relationship between the magnitude of Ppa rise and the fall in end-inspiratory Ppl seen in this study is that both changes were caused by lung hyperinflation and increased P$_A$. Elevated P$_A$ requires more negative Ppl to generate inspiratory airflow—and increased P$_A$ elevates intraluminal Ppa.

Effects of Pleural Pressure on Venous Return and Cardiac Output

Under steady state conditions, cardiac output (CO) equals venous return (VR) to the right heart. Since flow is determined by the pressure gradient across a system divided by flow resistance, VR is determined by dividing the difference between the driving pressure, referred to as mean systemic pressure (MSP), and the back pressure, which is generally considered to be right atrial pressure (Pra) by the resistance to venous return[29,30]:

$$VR = (MSP\text{-}Pra)/Rv \qquad (1)$$

When VR is plotted against Pra (Figure 3), the slope of the relationship reflects Rv. As Pra increases for any given Rv, VR decreases, approaching zero as Pra approaches MSP. Conversely, as Pra decreases, VR increases. At low levels of Pra (likely subatmospheric) flow is limited by the collapse of the great veins as they enter the thorax. Under these conditions, the back pressure is no longer Pra but the pressure surrounding the great vessels (Ps) and further decreases in Pra do not augment flow. As also seen in Fig-

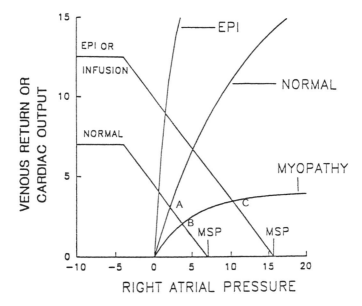

Figure 3. Venous return (VR) (or cardiac output) curves and cardiac function curves plotted against right atrial pressure (Pra). The slope of the relationship between VR and Pra is-1/Rv. As Pra increases for any given Rv, VR decreases, approaching zero as Pra approaches MSP. Conversely, as Pra decreases, VR increases. At low levels of Pra (about -4 cmH$_2$O in this figure) flow is limited by the collapse of the great veins as they enter the thorax. Under these conditions, the back pressure is no longer Pra but the pressure surrounding the great vessels and further decreases in Pra do not augment flow. The point of intersection between the venous return curves and the cardiac function curves represents steady state conditions (the Pra where VR equals CO). Point A represents the normal state. Note how VR or CO drops in myopathy (point A to point B), and how CO may be restored (point C) by increasing mean systemic pressure (MSP) with volume infusion or epinephrine. If epinephrine also shifts the cardiac function curve leftward CO will increase even further. (Modified from Scharf SM. Cardiopulmonary interactions. In: Scharf SM (ed). Cardiopulmonary Physiology in Critical Care. New York, NY, Marcel Dekker, Inc., 1992, p.155, with permission).

ure 3, VR increases at any given Pra when MSP increases (or when Rv decreases—not shown in Figure 3).

If cardiac function curves are plotted simultaneously with venous return curves (Figure 3), the point of intersection of the two curves represents steady state conditions (the Pra where VR equals CO). By way of example, note how VR or CO is maintained in the setting of reduced cardiac function by increasing MSP with volume infusion.

Because the right atrium is a flexible, compliant chamber, Pra is affected by changes in Ppl. During normal inspiration, the modest decrease in Ppl tends to increase VR by lowering Pra. In SA, the inspiratory large drop in Ppl (-20 to -40 cmH$_2$O) also lowers Pra and augments VR. However, VR is limited by collapse of extrathoracic veins at Pra below -4 to -8 cm H$_2$O.[31] Consistent with this physiology, Natori and coworkers[32] demonstrated a collapsed segment in the inferior vena cava (IVC) just below the diaphragm in asthmatics. Similarly, Nakhjavan and coworkers[33] demonstrated that at very high lung volumes in emphysema, the diaphragm may act as a sphincter on the IVC.

Because Ppl falls more during inspiration than it rises during expiration, mean Ppl decreases in spontaneously breathing asthmatics (even though there is prolongation of the expiratory phase).[25] This increases VR to the right heart, but compression of the IVC and increased Rv have the opposite effect. On balance, it appears that in non-intubated patients with SA, CO is slightly higher than normal.[26]

Despite enhanced VR to the right heart during inspiration, pulmonary artery blood flow does not increase during this phase of the respiratory cycle. Support for this statement again comes from Jardin and coworkers[25] and their study of PP in SA. In this study, the authors measured pulmonary artery and esophageal pressures in nine adults with SA and a PP of > 20 cmH$_2$O. Simultaneous two-dimensional echocardiography allowed for assessment of conformational changes in right and left heart chamber size throughout the respiratory cycle. Specifics regarding changes in Ppl and transmural systolic and diastolic pulmonary artery pressures are found above. Because there was a greater increase in diastolic pressure than in systolic pressure during inspiration, pulmonary artery pulse pressure (systolic pressure minus diastolic pressure)—which estimates stroke volume—decreased by about 3 mmHg. This suggests pulmonary blood flow did not increase during inspiration despite increased VR (assuming heart rate did not change significantly). Also, the increase in pulmonary artery diastolic pressure is consistent with increased PVR. Consistent with hemodynamic findings, echocardiographic data demonstrated that during inspiration there was an increase in end-systolic and end-diastolic right ventricular internal diameter. A likely explanation for these findings is that during inhalation PVR increased even further, increasing impedance to right ventricular ejection, and that increased RV preload and RV afterload increased RV dimensions throughout the cardiac cycle.

Wide swings in Ppl and Jardin's data help explain the phenomenon of PP in SA. PP is the difference between maximum and minimum systolic arterial blood pressure during the respiratory cycle. In SA, PP is greater than the normal value of 4 to 10 mmHg and is typically > 15 mmHg. As we have reviewed above, when Ppl falls during inspiration there is increased filling of the right atrium and right ventricle. The associated rise in lung volume increases PVR and right ventricular afterload. The combination of increased RV preload and RV afterload increases end-systolic and end-diastolic right ventricular internal diameter and shifts the intraventricular septum toward the left ventricle (LV). This conformational change in the LV (which results in diastolic dysfunction of that chamber) along with decreased RV stroke volume results in incomplete filling of the LV and decreased LV stroke volume. Additionally, large negative Ppl may directly impair LV emptying by increasing LV afterload.[34–36] Conversely, early in expiration, Ppl increases and lung volume decreases. Right ventricular afterload is reduced and RV stroke volume and LV filling increase. The intraventricular septum returns to a more normal position and LV stroke volume and systemic blood pressure temporarily increase. As expiration continues and Ppl increases further, RV preload drops and right ventricular stroke volume again begins to fall.

Effects of Cardiac Output on Pulmonary Artery Pressure

Whether the mild net increase in CO in patients with SA elevates Ppa is not known. In normals, increasing CO has little effect on Ppa. On the other hand, in patients with emphysema and destruction of the vascular bed, small increases in pulmonary blood flow, such as occur during exercise, can cause pulmonary hypertension.[37] In asthma, it is conceivable that functional obliteration of alveolar vessels by lung hyperinflation and increased P_A mimics the emphysematous state and accentuates the effects of increased CO on Ppa. Since the pulmonary circulation is essentially a collection of collapsible vessels, P_A affects the outflow or back pressure of this system (which is generally Pla). When Ppa is greater than Pla, and Pla is greater than P_A, (Zone III conditions) the driving pressure for blood flow is Ppa–Pla. However, if P_A exceeds Pla, (Zone II conditions), P_A becomes the effective outflow pressure, because the vessel exposed to P_A is compressed. Now the driving pressure is Ppa–P_A and further decreases in Pla do not influence flow. If P_A exceeds Ppa and Pla (Zone I conditions), there is no blood flow through the compressed vessel. In severe states of lung hyperinflation characterized by an increase in Zone 1 conditions, fewer blood vessels are available to accept the flow of blood through pulmonary circulation (i.e., functional obliteration of vasculature).

Effects of Positive Pressure Ventilation

Compared with spontaneously breathing patients, mechanically ventilated patients with SA are at increased risk of systemic hypotension, pneumothorax, and pulmonary hypertension because positive pressure ventilation may result in dangerous levels of lung hyperinflation.[38,39] During inspiration, Ppl and Pra increase to reduce VR to the right heart. At the same time positive pressure ventilation and lung inflation increase PVR and right ventricular afterload. The combination of decreased RV preload and increased RV afterload lowers RV stroke volume and LV filling.

In the post-intubation period, dangerous levels of lung hyperinflation can develop if patients are ventilated excessively. With severe airflow obstruction, even the delivery of a reduced minute ventilation (VE) can cause substantial gas trapping—increasing the risk of pneumothorax and hemodynamic compromise. When there is significant lung hyperinflation, inspired breaths are difficult to deliver (due to both airway obstruction and hyperinflation), breath sounds are diminished and neck veins are distended. Systemic blood pressure and pulse pressure fall, and pulse rate rises. These effects are accentuated by hypovolemia from increased insensible water losses and/or decreased oral fluid intake, sedation, and muscle relaxation—all of which decrease MSP and thus VR to the right heart. This pathophysiology can be demonstrated by hypoventilating the patient. Hypoventilation prolongs expiratory time and allows for greater lung emptying. This reduces mean intrathoracic pressure, increases blood pressure, increases pulse pressure, and decreases pulse rate (see below for specific recommendations regarding ventilator settings).

Effects of Arterial Blood Gases

Patients in SA often exhibit hypoxemia due to obstruction of peripheral airways and ventilation/perfusion mismatch (low V/Q). True shunt is minimal so correction of hypoxemia requires only modest enrichment of inspired oxygen (1-3 L/min by nasal cannula). McFadden and colleagues[40] found only 5% of acute asthmatics younger than age 45 had an initial PaO_2 of 55 mmHg or less at low altitude, suggesting that supplemental oxygen is not needed in the majority of cases. In this study, McFadden[40] also demonstrated a rough correlation between the degree of airflow obstruction as measured by the FEV_1 or PEFR and hypoxemia.

Alveolar hypoxia effectively vasoconstricts arterioles in the pulmonary circulation of normal subjects and in patients with lung disease. Hypoxic pulmonary vasoconstriction (HPV) decreases perfusion to poorly ventilated airspaces and helps to maintain normal V/Q ratios and PaO_2.[41] In patients with COPD, hypoxemia is associated with a rise in Ppa.[42] Supplemental oxygen produces a variable and often minimal fall in Ppa indicating that other factors are contributing to the development of pulmonary hypertension in these patients.[43]

Although the clinical significance of HPV in SA is not known, it is likely to be one of the factors responsible for the development of pulmonary hypertension in this condition. Accordingly, reversal of HPV with supplemental oxygen may lower Ppa. Oxygen may also reduce hyperpnea and thereby decrease lung inflation and PVR on that basis. Other benefits to oxygen include improved oxygen delivery to peripheral tissues (including respiratory muscles) and protection against the modest fall in PaO_2 often seen after administration of beta-agonists—which may vasodilate the pulmonary circulation and increase blood flow to low V/Q units.[44,45]

Respiratory alkalosis is common in the early stages of SA. If present for hours to days, respiratory alkalosis may induce compensatory renal bicarbonate wasting, which may manifest later as a non-anion gap metabolic acidosis. As the severity of airflow obstruction increases, $PaCO_2$ generally increases due to patient exhaustion and inadequate minute ventilation, and/or an increase in physiologic dead space. Patients with severe airflow obstruction may also develop an anion gap acidosis from accumulation of lactic acid.

In patients with COPD, there is a positive correlation between $PaCO_2$ and Ppa.[43] The mechanism whereby this effect occurs is not known. Harris and colleagues[18] speculated that hypercapnea induces hyperventilation, and that in patients with obstructive lung disease, this hyperventilation increases lung volume and PVR to elevate Ppa. In animal models, hypercapnea also constricts airways, but in humans, findings have been inconsistent.[46] Hypercapnea also potentiates HPV.[47] Hypercapnea may also have a direct effect on the pulmonary vasculature leading to pulmonary hypertension and an increase in end-systolic and end-diastolic RV volumes,[48] although this effect is likely minimal since hypercapnea generally increases CO.[49] Hypercapnea may also decrease myocardial contractility.[46]

Acute acidemia increases Ppa in normal subjects,[50] but has a variable effect on patients with COPD,[44] and an unknown effect in SA. However, acidemia likely augments the effects of hypoxia to produce pulmonary vasoconstriction.[43]

Effects of Mediators of Pulmonary Vasomotor Tone

Many naturally occurring substances have been shown to act as vasoconstrictors or vasodilators of the pulmonary circulation. But since most of the studies of these humoral substances have been performed in animals, extreme caution is warranted when translating these results to the human circulation.[14] Whether imbalances of such naturally occurring humoral substances in SA contributes to pulmonary vasoconstriction and the development of pulmonary hypertension in SA is not known. Some of these substances, such as catecholamines and histamine, increase PVR in man.[51] Serotonin, which may be elevated in some patients with SA, produces pulmonary vasoconstriction in animals but does not appear to do so in man.[51] Prostaglandins of the F series may cause vasoconstriction whereas prostaglandins of the E series result in vasoconstriction.

Summary of Factors Contributing to Pulmonary Hypertension in Status Asthmaticus

As evident in the previous sections, it is likely that several different mechanisms underlie the development of pulmonary hypertension in patients with SA. Chief among these, however, seems to be lung hyperinflation, which is the result of expiratory airflow obstruction and hyperpnea. Lung hyperinflation increases PVR by compressing alveolar vessels, and may also (at least theoretically) restrict the movement of the walls of the cardiac fossa.

To overcome increased resistive and elastic loads, patients with SA generate significantly negative Ppl during inspiration. The drop in Ppl increases VR to the right heart, although this is somewhat offset by an increase in Rv resulting from lung hyperinflation and its affects on the great veins, and by positive Ppl during expiration. Whether this net increase in VR and CO elevates Ppa in SA is not known. It is conceivable that functional obliteration of alveolar vessels by lung hyperinflation accentuates the effects of increased CO on Ppa—analogous to what happens in patients with emphysema.

Alterations in arterial blood gases may contribute to pulmonary hypertension in SA. Hypoxic pulmonary vasoconstriction increases PVR and Ppa. This effect is augmented by hypercapnea and acidemia. Hypercapnea may also directly vasoconstrict the pulmonary circulation, or increase PVR by inducing hyperventilation and worsening lung hyperinflation.

Finally, it is possible that changes in naturally occurring humoral substances, such as catecholamines, histamine, and prostaglandins contribute to pulmonary vasoconstriction and the development of pulmonary hypertension in SA.

Implications for Treatment

In general, current therapeutic strategies in SA decrease lung hyperinflation and lead to correction of arterial blood gas abnormalities. This likely explains why signs and symptoms of pulmonary hypertension typically resolve within hours of successful treatment. Accordingly, routine asthma management is all that is required in most patients.

Pharmacologic Therapy

In most patients with SA, immediate treatment of airway smooth muscle mediated bronchoconstriction and airway wall inflammation with beta-agonists and corticosteroids, respectively, effectively decreases airflow obstruction. Anticholinergics play a lesser role in the treatment of acute asthma, and debate continues regarding the efficacy of theophylline in this setting. By decreasing airflow obstruction through pharmacologic means, expiratory airflow improves, and there is greater emptying of alveolar gas. At the same time, correction of arterial hypoxemia with supplemental oxygen reverses hypoxic pulmonary vasoconstriction and its contribution to higher Ppa.

Mechanical Ventilation

Patients failing drug therapy should be considered early for intubation and mechanical ventilation. A strategy of mechanical ventilation that prolongs expiratory time by limiting V_E and by decreasing inspiratory time decreases the risk of systemic hypotension, pneumothorax and pulmonary hypertension, and should improve the outcome of these most critically ill asthmatics. Ventilator-applied PEEP should be avoided because it has the potential to increase lung volume.[52]

For an average sized adult an initial V_E between 8 and 10 L/min combined with an inspiratory flow rate of 100 L/min is unlikely to result in a dangerous degree of lung hyperinflation.[53] One way to ensure that ventilator setting have not resulted in excessive air trapping is to collect the total exhaled volume during a period of apnea. This volume, termed by Tuxen[38] "V_{EI}", is the volume of gas at end-inspiration above FRC. A V_{EI} above 20 mL/kg (1.4 L in an average sized adult) has been shown to predict complications of hypotension and barotrauma.[53] Tuxen[38] has used V_{EI} to regulate V_E to a safe level (i.e, that not resulting in $V_{EI} > 20$ mL/kg) in ventilated asthmatics. Respiratory rate was decreased when V_{EI} was > 20 mL/kg, and increased when V_{EI} was < 20 mL/kg. At the beginning of mechanical ventilation, the safe level of V_E often resulted in hypercapnea, but as airflow obstruction improved, the V_E deemed safe approached the V_E required for normocapnea; and when safe V_E achieved a $PaCO_2 < 40$ mmHg, patients were evaluated for extubation. Alternatively, the static or plateau pressure on the ventilator, which is an estimate of average end-inspiratory alveolar pressures, may be used as a marker of lung inflation.[54]

Although permissive hypercapnea allows for less lung inflation, it is not without potential risk. As stated above, hypercapneic acidosis may, among other effects, decrease myocardial contractility and augment pulmonary vasoconstriction.[55] Still, permissive hypercapnea is well tolerated by many patients as long as $PaCO_2$ does not exceed 90 mmHg[56] and acute increases in $PaCO_2$ are avoided. Although further studies are needed regarding the risks and benefits of permissive hypercapnea, available data currently support a ventilatory strategy in SA that limits lung hyperinflation by permitting hypercapnea.[54]

References

1. American Thoracic Society. Standards for the diagnosis and care of patients with chronic obstructive pulmonary disease (COPD) and asthma. Am Rev Respir Dis 1987;136:225–244.
2. National Heart, Lung, and Blood Institute, National Asthma Education Program, Expert Panel Report. Guidelines for the diagnosis and management of asthma. J Allergy Clin Immunol 1991;88:425–433.
3. Grossman J. The occurrence of arrhythmias in hospitalized asthma patients. J Allergy Clin Immunol 1976;57:310–317.
4. Josephson GW, Kennedy HL, MacKenzie EJ, et al. Cardiac dysrhythmias during the treatment of acute asthma: A comparison of two treatment regimens by a double blind protocol. Chest 1980;78:429–35.
5. Scharf S. Mechanical cardiopulmonary interactions with asthma. Clin Rev Allergy 1985;3:487–500.
6. Rebuck AS, Read J. Assessment and management of severe asthma. Am J Med 1971;51:788–98.
7. Wasserfallen JB, Schaller MD, Feihl F, et al. Sudden asphyxic asthma: A distinct entity? Am Rev Respir Dis 1990;142:108–11.
8. Sur S, Crotty TB, Kephart GM, et at. Sudden-onset fatal asthma: A distinct clinical entity with few eosinophils and relatively more neutrophils in the airway submucosa. Am Rev Respir Dis 1993;148:713–19.
9. Ried LM. The presence or absence of bronchial mucus in fatal asthma. J Allergy Clin Immunol 1987;80:415–16.
10. Permutt S, Wise RA. Mechanical interaction of respiration and circulation. In: Fishman A (ed). Handbook of Physiology, volume 3. American Physiological Society, Baltimore, MD, Williams and Wilkins, 1986, p.647-656.
11. Permutt S, Howell JBL, Proctor DF, et al. Effects of lung inflation on static volume characteristics of pulmonary vessels. J Appl Physiol 1961;16:64–70.
12. Whittenberg JL, McGregor M, Berglund E, et al. Influence of state of inflation of the lung on pulmonary vascular resistance. J Appl Physiol 1960;15:878–82.
13. Roos A, Thomas LJ, Nagel EL, et al. Pulmonary vascular resistance as determined by lung inflation and vascular pressure. J Appl Physiol 1961;16:77–84.
14. Murray JF. Circulation. In: Murray JF (ed). The Normal Lung. The Basis for Diagnosis and Treatment of Pulmonary disease. Philadelphia, PA, W. B. Saunders Co., 1976 pp.113–150.
15. Pinsky MR. Determinants of pulmonary flow variation during respiration. J Appl Physiol 1984;56:1237–45.
16. Butler J, Paley HW. Lung volume and pulmonary circulation. Med Thorax 1962;19:261–67.

17. Canada E, Benumof JL, Tousdale FR. Pulmonary vascular resistance correlated in intact normal and abnormal canine lungs. Crit Care Med 1982;10:719–23.
18. Harris P, Segel N, Green I, et al. The influence of the airways resistance and alveolar pressure on the pulmonary vascular resistance in chronic bronchitis. Cardiovasc Res 1968;2:84–92.
19. Permut S. Relation between pulmonary artery pressure and pleural pressure during the acute asthmatic attack. Chest 1973;63(Suppl):25S–27S.
20. Permut S, Bromberger-Barnea B, Bane HN. Alveolar pressure, pulmonary venous pressure and the vascular waterfall. Med Thorac 1962;19:239–60.
21. Butler J. The heart is not always in good hands. Chest 1990;97:453–60.
22. Robertson CH, Hall DL, Hogg JC. A description of lung distortion due to localized pleural stress. J Appl Physiol 1973;34:344–50.
23. Freedman S, Tattersfield AE, Pride NB. Changes in lung mechanics during asthma induced by exercise. J Appl Physiol 1975;38:974–81.
24. Holmes PW, Campbell AH, Barter CE. Acute changes of lung volumes and lung mechanics in asthma and in normal subjects. Thorax 1978;33:394–400.
25. Stalcup SA, Mellins RB. Mechanical forces producing pulmonary edema in acute asthma. N Engl J Med 1977;297:592–96.
26. Jardin F, Farcot, JC, Boisante L, et al. Mechanism of paradoxic pulse in bronchial asthma. Circulation 1982;66:887–94.
27. O'Quin R, Marini JJ. Pulmonary artery occlusion pressure: Clinical physiology, measurement, and interpretation. Am Rev Resp Dis 1983;128:319–26.
28. Gunstone RF: Right heart pressures in bronchial asthma. Thorax 1971;26:39–45.
29. Goldberg HS, Rabson J. Control of cardiac output by systemic vessels: Circulatory adjustments to acute and chronic respiratory failure and the effect of therapeutic interventions. Am J Cardiol 1981;47:696–702.
30. Scharf SM. Cardiopulmonary interactions. In: Scharf SM (ed). Cardiopulmonary Physiology in Critical Care. New York, Marcel Dekker, Inc., 1992, pp.333–355.
31. Brecher GA. Mechanism of venous flow under different degrees of aspiration. Am J Physiol 1952;169:423–33.
32. Natori H, Tamaki S, Dira S. Ultrasonographic evaluation of ventilatory effect on inferior cava configuration. Am Rev Respir Dis 1979;120:421–27.
33. Nakhjavan FK, Palmer WH, McGregor M. Influence of respiration on venous return in emphysema. Circulation 1966;33:8–16.
34. Scharf S, Brown R, Sounders N, et al. Effects of normal and loaded spontaneous inspiration on cardiovascular function. J Appl Physiol 1979;47:582–90.
35. Scharf S, Brown R, Tow D, et al. Cardiac effects of increased lung volume and decreased pleural pressure. J Appl Physiol 1979;47:257–62.
36. Buda AJ, Pinsky MR, Ingels NB Jr, et al. Effect of intrathoracic pressure on left ventricular performance. N Engl J Med 1979;301:453–59.
37. Matthay RA, Niederman MS, Weideman HP. Cardiovascular-pulmonary interaction in chronic obstructive pulmonary disease with special attention reference to the pathogenesis and management of core pulmonale. Med Clin North Am 1990;74:571–618.
38. Tuxen DV, Williams TJ, Scheinkestel CD, et al. Use of a measurement of pulmonary hyperinflation to control the level of mechanical ventilation in patients with acute severe asthma. Am Rev Respir Dis 1992;146:1136–42.
39. Tuxen DV, Lane S. The effects of ventilatory pattern on hyperinflation, airway pressures, and circulation in mechanical ventilation of patients with severe airflow obstruction. Am Rev Respir Dis 1987;136:872–79.

40. McFadden ER Jr, Lyons HA. Arterial-blood gas tension in asthma. N Engl J Med 1968;278:1027–32.
41. Fishman AP. Hypoxia and its effects on the pulmonary circulation. How and where it acts. Circ Res 1979;38:221–31.
42. Bishop JM, Cross KW. Use of physiological variables to predict pulmonary artery pressure in patients with chronic respiratory disease-a multicentre study. Eur Heart J 1981;2:509–17.
43. Macnee W. Pathophysiology of cor pulmonale in chronic obstructive pulmonary disease: part one. State of the art. Am J Resp Crit Care Med 1994;150: 833–52.
44. West JB: State of the art: Ventilation-perfusion relationships. Am Rev Respir Dis 1977;116:919–43.
45. Ballester E, Reyes A, Roca J, et al. Ventilation-perfusion mismatching in acute severe asthma: effects of salbutamol and 100% oxygen. Thorax 1989;44:258–67.
46. Feihl F, Perret C: Persmissive hypercapnia: how permissive should we be? State of the art. Am J Resp Crit Care Med 1994;150:1722–37.
47. Durand J, Leroy-Ladurie M, Ransom-Bitker B. Effects of hypoxia and hypercapnia on the repartition of pulmonary blood flow insupine subjects. Progress in Resp Research 1970;5:156–65.
48. Viitianen A, Salmenpera M, Heinonen J. Right ventricular response to hypercapnia after cardiac surgery. Anesthesiology 1990;73:393–400.
49. Kilburn KH, Asmundsson T, Britt RC, et al. Effects of breathing 10% carbon dioxide on the pulmonary circulation of human subjects. Circulation 1969;39: 639–53.
50. Aber GM, Bayley TJ, Bishop JM. Inter-relationship between renal and cardiac function and respiratory gas exchange in obstructive airways disease. Clin Sci 1963;25:159–70.
51. Dollery CT, Glazier JB. Pharmacological effects of drugs on the pulmonary circulation in man. Clin Pharmacol Ther 1966;7:807–18.
52. Tuxen DV. Detrimental effects of positive end-expiratory pressure during controlled mechanical ventilation of patients with severe airflow obstruction. Am Rev Respir Dis 1989;140:5–9.
53. Williams TJ, Tuxen DV, Scheinkestel CD, et al. Risk factors for morbidity in mechanically ventilated patients with acute severe asthma. Am Rev Respir Dis 1992;146:607–15.
54. Corbridge T, Hall JB. The assessment and management of adults with status asthmaticus. State of the art. Am J Resp Crit Care Med 1994.
55. Tuxen DV: Permissive hypercapnic ventilation. Am J Respir Crit Care Med 1994;150:870–74.
56. Darioli R, Perret C. Mechanical controlled hypoventilation in status asthmaticus. Am Rev Respir Dis 1984;129:385–87.
57. Corbridge T, Irvin CG. Pathophysiology of chronic obstructive pulmonary disease with emphasis on physiologic and pathologic correlations. In: Casaburi R, Petty T (eds). Principles and Practice of Pulmonary Rehabilitation. Philadelphia, PA, W. B. Saunders Co., 1993, pp. 18–32.

Chapter 7

Cor Pulmonale

Part I

Anthony M. Cosentino, M.D.

Definition

Ask a medical student or house officer the definition of cor pulmonale and the usual response is that it is right heart failure secondary to pulmonary disease. Inquire further as to how they diagnose the presence of heart failure and they will usually site the onset of peripheral edema.

The generally accepted definition of cor pulmonale is right ventricular (RV) enlargement and/or right ventricular hypertrophy (RVH) secondary to pulmonary disease and absent left ventricular (LV) failure.[1] Fortunately, the presence of right heart failure is not required for the diagnosis, since we will see that the criteria for the presence of right heart failure are infrequently present.

Diagnosis

The diagnosis of cor pulmonale as with any diagnosis begins with history, but except for a history of pre-existing lung disease, it is rarely helpful in ascertaining the point at which RVH supervenes. However, a decrease in exercise tolerance and general deterioration in a patient with stable chronic obstructive pulmonary disease (COPD), i.e., stable forced expiratory volume in 1 second and arterial blood gases, may be a harbinger of cardiovascular dysfunction.

From: Cosentino AM, Martin RJ (eds.): Cardiothoracic Interrelationships in Clinical Practice. © Futura Publishing Co., Inc., Armonk, NY, 1997.

The physical examination proves to be almost as unrewarding. An elevated jugular venous pressure must be interpreted relative to intrapleural pressures. In pulmonary emphysema with loss of lung elasticity, pleural pressure (P_{Pl}) at functional residual capacity (FRC) may be significantly more positive than normal, and in pulmonary fibrosis with increase in elastic recoil P_{Pl} will be more negative at FRC.

Palpation of the chest may reveal an RV heave but this finding is usually obscured by lung hyperinflation in COPD. A prominent pulsation below the xiphisternum may provide a clue as to the presence of RVH but the sensitivity and specificity of this finding has never been evaluated. An S_4 audible in this area may, however, strongly suggest the diagnosis, especially if the loudness increases with inspiration. A murmur of tricuspid insufficiency in my experience is heard only infrequently. The classic changes in the second heart sound associated with decreased pulmonary vascular capacitance are an increase in the second component and a narrowing of the split, which remains fixed. Again in my experience except for pulmonary thromboembolic disease this sign is elicited only infrequently.

Chest x rays may be helpful. Matthay and coworkers reported that the diameter of the descending branch of the pulmonary artery (PA) was >16 mm in 43 of 46 patients with pulmonary hypertension.[2] Chetty and colleagues[3] found that specificity for a diagnosis of pulmonary hypertension was better served if we demand that the descending branch of the right PA be >20 mm. They also reported that an increase in the hilar cardiothoracic ratio had a sensitivity of 95% and a specificity of 100% for the presence of pulmonary hypertension in patients with COPD. However, since the subjects are preselected, i.e., have COPD, what in fact is being reported is the negative and positive predictive values of that criterion rather than sensitivity and specificity.

In fact, in the usual clinical circumstance the diagnosis is most frequently based on the ECG. It is sometimes forgotten that patients chosen for studies of the ECG in pulmonary disease were chosen on clinical criteria, so that data on sensitivity and specificity are difficult to obtain. Nevertheless, Spodick[4] concluded that the verticality of the P vector (between +70 and +90) was the most distinctive finding. He also noted gothic P waves in II, III, AVF, and diphasic P waves in the precordial leads. The majority of his patients had COPD.[5] Data on sensitivity and specificity has been lacking. In fact, a recent publication showed a lack of correlation between P pulmonale and right atrial (RA) overload in COPD.[5] All patients with P pulmonale showed impaired lung function but almost all had "normal" hemodynamic function, i.e., normal RA and PA pressures. They also concluded that verticalization of the heart, especially vertical extension of the right atrium, seemed to be a more likely and a more important factor for P pulmonale in COPD than the hemodynamic effects of impaired lung function on the right atrium.

Butler et al.,[6] in a study of mitral stenosis, introduced three criteria for RVH: (1) P wave amplitude >0.25 mV in leads II, III, and AVF, V_1, or V_2; (2) R wave amplitude <0.2 mV in lead I; and (3) A + R + PL >0.7 mV (A = R or R_1 in V_1 or V_2; R = S in I or V_6; PL = S in V_2).

Behar et al.,[7] studied these criteria in mitral stenosis and cor pulmonale and reported that in cor pulmonale, these criteria achieved a sensitivity of 89%.

A recent report from Japan showed that P pulmonale was infrequent with pulmonary fibrosis and that while the P wave axis was usually > +70 in COPD it was invariably < +70 in pulmonary fibrosis.[8] They concluded that the P wave axis correlated with hyperinflation rather than with R atrial hypertension.

Another publication[9] suggests that the esophageal ECG is much more sensitive and accurate than the routine ECG in diagnosing RVH in cases of COPD. Clearly this is not a practical screening procedure in the evaluation of such patients, but certainly serves to demonstrate the difficulties inherent in the diagnosis of cor pulmonale.

Himmelman et al.,[10] at UCSF, studied the two-dimensional echocardiogram with Doppler analysis in 33 patients with COPD. Tricuspid regurgitation was studied by injection of agitated saline and RA pressure was estimated by sonospirometry. Only patients with a PaO_2 >55 mmHg were studied. Sleeping oximetry was also performed. Of these patients, only one had RVH by ECG criteria, and by examination nine had RVH or failure. Overall, 13 had clinical evidence of cor pulmonale. Nocturnal desaturation did not explain the occurrence of cor pulmonale. Pulmonary hypertension was present in 16 patients. Overall, 76% had evidence of cor pulmonale by echocardiography versus 39% by clinical methods.

Because "pulmonary arterial hypertension cannot be reliably recognized nor its degree of severity determined by clinical methods alone," a multicenter study was designed to develop research into these problems.[11] In COPD, of the physiologic variables studied, the best correlation was found with arterial oxygen saturation. Though the precision of the prediction of mean PA pressure was high for the group of COPD patients studied, prediction of PA pressure in any one individual was not possible with any degree of accuracy. Curiously in fibrosing alveolitis, mild to moderate degrees of hypoxemia were more frequently associated with pulmonary hypertension than in the other groups studied.

Clearly, the diagnosis of pulmonary hypertension and/or cor pulmonale is difficult. Good data on sensitivity, specificity, and positive and negative predictive values is lacking.

Pathology

One might reasonably ask if there is a gold standard for the diagnosis of cor pulmonale. The thickness of the RV is widely used by pathologists as an index of RVH. Mitchell et al.,[12] found a correlation between RV thickness and weight that was significant (r = 0.65) but the relationship was poor in a number of cases. They chose to use RV weight as a criterion for RVH but found comparable to the findings of others that the correlation of RV weight with degree of emphysema is weak. Curiously this correlation improved in that subset of patients with large airways disease but normal small airways.

They did find an excellent correlation between RV weights and the ECG diagnosis of cor pulmonale in those patients with COPD (85% sensitivity).

Pathophysiology

Cor pulmonale is generally assumed to be secondary to pulmonary hypertension and pulmonary hypertension is generally assumed to be secondary to hypoxic pulmonary vasoconstriction. There is a paucity of data to support these notions and in fact, autopsy data shows a poor correlation between PA pressure and RVH.[13] The previous lack of correlation between P pulmonale and RA overload has been referred to. Might this discrepancy be explained if we studied PA pressure relative to intrapleural pressure? This is addressed further in Chapter 6 where we explore cor pulmonale in asthma. At this point it is sufficient to appreciate that intrapleural pressures will vary significantly dependent upon the disease state, i.e., asthma or emphysema. In Himmelman's study,[10] RA pressure determined by sonospirometry was normal in four-fifths of their patients and in fact varied from 2.5–17.5 mmHg. Intrapleural pressures were not evaluated and patients were not separated into COPD subsets.

Even more elementary is the mechanism of pulmonary hypertension. The pulmonary vascular bed is a high capacitance bed and can accommodate a fourfold increase in flow without an increase in PA pressure and states of increased flow such as atrial septal defects can be tolerated for many years without development of increased vascular resistance.

Wright, Petty, and Thurlbeck[14] studied the pulmonary vascular anatomy at necropsy in patients with COPD enrolled in the National Institutes of Health nocturnal oxygen therapy trial. They found structural alterations of the muscular pulmonary arteries, which consisted of markedly increased percentages of intima and media, most pronounced in medium and larger muscular arteries. However, these changes did not correlate with either the severity of the pulmonary hypertension or the ability of the pulmonary vasculature to respond to oxygen administration.

It is often stated that the vascular changes are secondary to hypoxic vasoconstriction. Wilkinson et al.[15] examined the pulmonary vascular structure in patients treated with and without O_2 and found no difference in those treated or not treated. They found marked intimal proliferation with normal or atrophic muscular media in the muscular arteries, associated with extension of muscle into the arterioles.

It would appear that although cor pulmonale in COPD is associated with hypoxemia that hypoxic vasoconstriction alone cannot explain the physiologic and pathologic alterations seen in patients with pulmonary vascular alteration secondary to COPD.

Block and colleagues[16] have suggested that nocturnal oxygen desaturation may explain many cases of pulmonary hypertension unassociated with significant daytime hypoxemia. Clearly in the British long-term O_2 in COPD study, nocturnal oxygen did ameliorate pulmonary hypertension.[17] However, it should be noted that their subjects had significantly more severe pulmonary hypertension than subjects enrolled in the American study.[18] Mean PA pressures were 42.5 before O_2 and 32.3 mmHg after prolonged O_2. Also, the hematocrit decreased from 51.4% to 42.5%. These data may suggest that polycythemia is a good predictor of who will benefit most from nocturnal O_2. The results in the American study were much less dramatic.[19]

Herles et al.,[20] in attempt to delineate the site of increased pulmonary vascular resistance (PVR) in cor pulmonale, noted a "significant relation" between the PA wedge pressure and the PA pressure. In uncomplicated chronic bronchitis, the PA wedge pressure was never raised. In cor pulmonale with "heart failure," it was raised in more than half and after treatment remained elevated in 20%.

Harris et al.,[21] in 1968, addressed the possibility that pulmonary hypertension was related to the influence of airways resistance and alveolar pressure on PVR in COPD. They were the first to demonstrate an increase in wedge pressure with resting hyperventilation in COPD.

Butler et al.[22] confirmed these findings and demonstrated lower lobe gas trapping. RA pressures also increased similar to the increase in wedge pressure and thus they concluded that the increase in wedge pressure was due to an increase in juxtacardiac pressure secondary to lower lobe hyperinflation.

A further puzzle is the apparent increase in PVR with exercise in COPD.[22–24] In subjects with stable COPD, i.e., without evidence of cor pulmonale, this may be related to the assumption that the pressure-flow relationship is a straight line and passes through zero. We saw in Chapter 1, Physiology, that this is not true. However, over the rectilinear portion of the curve, the slope is constant and thus resistance does not increase.[25] In patients with cor pulmonale, the increase in PA pressure is even more dramatic and since cardiac output (CO) increases very little, "resistance" rises dramatically[22] (Figures 1 and 2). The curious student must ask why? In stable COPD, the increase in PA pressure may be due to an increase in flow without an increase in PVR if we examine the rectilinear portion of the pressure-flow curve. However, in cor pulmonale, the increase in PA pressure greatly exceeds the increase in flow and clearly there is an increased impediment to flow. In light of the observations made, it seems reasonable to conclude that the increase in PVR and PA pressure with exercise, and the blunted cardiovascular response to exercise in cor pulmonale is a consequence of perturbations in lung and thoracic mechanics.

Finally, we must ask, "Does the RV fail?" If we diagnose RV failure as a decreased CO, the answer in most cases is no. Many series have reported normal or increased CO at rest and normal or decreased peripheral vascular resistance, contrary to the findings in LV failure.[26] However, as noted, the response of CO to exercise has been abnormal and has been interpreted as evidence for a failing RV.

The functional status of the RV in COPD with and without cor pul-

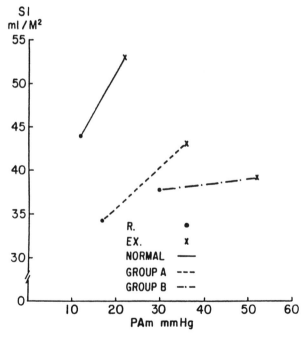

Figure 1. Stroke output in patients with chronic obstructive lung disease is significantly compromised secondary to the increased pressure work. PAm = pulmonary artery mean pressure; R = mean values at rest; Ex = mean values during exercise; SI = stroke index. (Reprinted with permission from Ref. 23.)

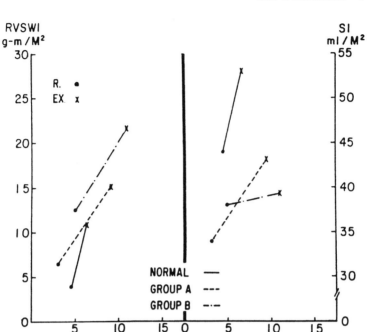

Figure 2. Right ventricular stroke work index (RVSWI) is highest in patients with cor pulmonale both at rest (R) and during exercise (Ex). All three groups form a single RV function curve, but patients with chronic obstructive lung disease operate on an extension of this curve with abdominal RVEDPs during exercise. However, when SI is related to the RVEDP, patients with cor pulmonale show depressed RV function. (Reprinted with permission from Ref. 23.)

monale has been a subject of significant interest and fraught with difficulties in interpretation. The blunted response in CO with exercise has been associated with an increase in right ventricular end-diastolic pressure (RVEDP). According to the Frank-Starling hypothesis, an increase in preload should be associated with an increase in CO. These observations would then suggest that the RV is failing. However, this ignores the effect of afterload on RV performance. Khaja and Parker[23] showed that although stroke index (SI) versus RVEDP was depressed, in fact stroke work was significantly increased and thus, RV function was concluded to be normal (Figures 1 and 2). This nicely demonstrates the difficulties in assessing myocardial contractility in the presence of an increase in afterload. Sagawa et al.[27] showed that the end-systolic pressure volume relation is a valid means of evaluating the functional status of the LV and that this method is independent of preload and afterload. MacNee[28] demonstrated that this technique was also valid in the evaluation of the contractility of the RV. Several studies utilizing this technique in COPD with pulmonary hypertension have documented normal, or even hypernormal, RV contractility.[29,30]

Another index of contractility, the maximal isovolumic rate of development of ventricular pressure has also been reported to be normal in COPD even with pulmonary hypertension.[31]

Because of the unique geometry of the RV, angiographic studies of RV ejection fraction have been difficult to interpret. This led to the use of radionuclide angiography. These studies may be summarized by saying that the mean RV ejection fraction in most subjects with COPD is lower than normal, but there is considerable overlap with normal. RV ejection fraction measured with this technique in cor pulmonale with edema has been moderately reduced and again the normal increase in right ventricular ejection fraction (RVEF) with exercise does not occur.[32] These data must be interpreted in the presence of increased RV afterload.

In summary, in patients with COPD without cor pulmonale CO is normal at rest and the response to exercise is blunted. However, the relationship of oxygen consumption to CO remains normal and it may be concluded that the primary limitation to exercise is pulmonary. Indices of RV contractility have been normal.

Pulmonary hypertension tends to be only moderate, but may rise appreciably with exercise, particularly in subjects with cor pulmonale. PVR appears to increase significantly but may in part be related to assumptions that render the calculated values misleading. Further, the wedge pressure may rise and further alterations in lung mechanics may, in fact, alter the geometry of the intraparenchymal pulmonary vasculature.

In subjects with cor pulmonale, RV ejection fraction measured by radionuclide angiography is often modestly reduced. However, stroke work index and other indices of contractility remain normal. CO is normal or increased at rest but rises little with exercise.

In subjects with cor pulmonale and edema, CO remains normal though the end-systolic pressure volume ratio may be lower than in stable COPD.

The mechanism of edema formation will be examined in Chapter 7, Part II.

Left Ventricle in Cor Pulmonale

As many as 30% of patients with COPD at autopsy have been reported to have LV hypertrophy.[33–35] Whether this is secondary to COPD and/or cor pulmonale or due to other diseases that may affect the left ventricle is controversial.[36,37] Most studies have shown a normal LV ejection fraction at rest[23] but results during exercise have been variable.[23,38,39] As noted previously, increased LV filling pressures have been noted during exercise[38,39] but may be related to changes in lung mechanics as described by both Harris and Butler, and previously noted in this chapter. The markedly negative swings in intrapleural pressure seen in COPD, particularly during exercise could also affect the left ventricle as a result of the resultant increase in LV transmural pressure and thus an increase in LV afterload.[40] However, it is extremely unusual to see clinical evidence of LV dysfunction. Systemic peripheral vascular resistance, regularly elevated in LV failure is decreased or normal in cor pulmonale. Also, pulmonary plethora and pleural effusions are not seen in the absence of other causes of LV dysfunction or mitral valve disease.

References

1. World Health Organization. Chronic cor pulmonale: A report of the expert committee. Circulation 1963;27:594–598.
2. Matthay RA, Schwarz MI, Ellis JH Jr, et al. Pulmonary artery hypertension in chronic obstructive pulmonary disease: Chest radiographic assessment. Invest Radiol 1981;16:95–100.
3. Chetty KG, Brown SE, White RW. Identification of pulmonary hypertension in chronic obstructive pulmonary disease from routine chest radiographs. Am Rev Respir Dis 1982;126:338–341.
4. Spodick DH. Electrocardiographic studies in pulmonary disease. Circulation 1959;20:1067–1074.
5. Maeda S, Hideki K, Kouji C, et al. Lack of correlation between P pulmonale and right atrial overload in chronic obstructive airways disease. Br Heart J 1991; 65:132–136.
6. Butler PM, Leggett SI, Howe CM, et al. Identification of electrocardiographic criteria for diagnosis of right ventricular hypertrophy due to mitral stenosis. Am J Cardiol 1986;57:639–643.
7. Behar JV, Howe CM, Wagner MB, et al. Performance of new criteria for right ventricular hypertrophy and myocardial infarction in patients with pulmonary hypertension due to cor pulmonale and mitral stenosis. J Electrocardiol 1991; 24:231–237.
8. Ikeda K, Kubota I, Takahashi K, et al. P wave changes in obstructive and restrictive lung diseases. J Electrocardiol 1985;18:233–238.
9. Mittal SR, Jain SC, Sharma SK. Esophageal ECG is more sensitive and accurate than the routine ECG in diagnosing RVH in cases of COPD. Int J Cardiol 1986;11:165–173.
10. Himmelman RB, Struve SN, Brown JK, et al. Improved recognition of cor pulmonale in patients with severe chronic obstructive pulmonary disease. Am J Med 1988;84:891–898.
11. Bishop JM, Cross KW. Use of other physiological variables to predict pulmonary arterial pressure in patients with COPD: Multicenter study. Eur Heart J 1981;2: 509–517.

12. Mitchell RS, Standford RE, Silvers GW, et al. The right ventricular and chronic airway obstruction: A clinical pathologic study. Am Rev Respir Dis 1976;114: 147–154.
13. Lehtonen J, Sutinen S, Ikaheimo P, et al. Electrocardiographic criteria for the diagnosis of right ventricular hypertrophy verified at autopsy. Chest 1988;93: 839–842.
14. Wright JL, Petty T, Thurlbeck WM. Analysis of the structure of the muscular pulmonary arteries in patients with pulmonary hypertension and COPD: National institutes of health nocturnal oxygen therapy trial. Lung 1992;170:109–124.
15. Wilkinson M, Langhorne CA, Heath D, et al. A pathophysiological study of 10 cases of hyposic cor pulmonale. Q J Med 1988;249:65–85.
16. Block AJ, Boysen PG, Wynee JW: The origins of cor pulmonale. A hypothesis. Chest 1968;75:147–156.
17. Abraham AS, Cole RB, Bishop JM. Reversal of pulmonary hypertension by prolonged O_2 administration to patients with chronic bronchitis. Circ Res 1968;23: 147–156.
18. Nocturnal Oxygen Therapy Trial Group. Continuous or nocturnal oxygen therapy in high toxemic COLD. Ann Intern Med 1980;92:391–398.
19. Timms RM, Khaja FU, William GW. The Nocturnal Oxygen Therapy Trial Group: Hemodynamic response to oxygen therapy in COPD. Ann Intern Med 1985;102:29–36.
20. Herles F, Jezek V, Daum S. Site of pulmonary resistance in cor pulmonale in chronic bronchitis. Br Heart J 1968;30:654–660.
21. Harris P, Segel N, Green J, et al. The influence of the airways resistance and alveolar pressure on the pulmonary vascular resistance in chronic bronchitis. Cardiovasc Res 1968;2:84–94.
22. Butler J, Schrijen F, Henriquez A, et al. Cause of the raised wedge pressure on exercise in chronic obstructive pulmonary disease. Am Rev Respir Dis 1988; 138:350–354.
23. Khaja F, Parker JO. Right and left ventricular performance in chronic obstructive lung disease. Am Heart J 1971;83:319–327.
24. Matthay RA, Arroliga AC, Wiedemann HP, et al. Right ventricular function at rest and during exercise in chronic obstructive pulmonary disease. Chest 1992; 101:255S–262S.
25. Graham R, Skoog C, Matthido W, et al. Dopamine, dobutamine, and phentolamine effects on pulmonary vascular mechanics. J Appl Physiol 1983;54: 1277–1283.
26. Fishman AP. State of the art: Chronic cor pulmonale. Am Rev Respir Dis 1976; 114:775–794.
27. Sagawa K, Suga H, Shoukas AA, et al. Endsystolic pressure-volume ratio. A new index of contractility. Am J Cardiol 1977;40:748–753.
28. MacNee W. Right ventricular function in cor pulmonale. Cardiol 1988;75: S30–S40.
29. MacNee W, Wathen CG, Hannan WJ, et al. Effects of pirbuterol and sodium nitro prusside on pulmonary hemodynamics in hypoxic cor pulmonale. Br Med J 1983;287:1169–1172.
30. Biernacki W, Flenley CD, Muir AL, et al. Pulmonary hypertension and RV function in patients with COPD. Chest 1988;94:1169–1175.
31. Stein PD, Sabbah NH, Anbe DT, et al. Performance of the failing and non failing RV of patients with pulmonary hypertension. Am J Cardiol 1979;44: 1050–1055.

32. MacNee W. State of the art. Pathophysiology of cor pulmonale in COPD. Am J Respir Crit Care Med 1994;150(Part I):833–852.
33. Edwards CW. Left ventricular hypertrophy in emphysema. Thorax 1974;29: 75–80.
34. Fluck DC, Chandrasekar RG, Gardener FV. The ventricular hypertrophy in chronic bronchitis. Br Heart J 1966;28:92–97.
35. Kohama A, Tanouchi J, Masatsuga H, et al. Pathologic involvement of the left ventricle in chronic cor pulmonale. Chest 1990;98:794–800.
36. Lockhart A, Tzareva M, Nader F, et al. Elevated pulmonary—A wedge pressure at rest and during exercise in chronic bronchitis: Fact of fancy. Clin Sci 1969;37:503–517.
37. MacNee W. State of the art. Pathophysiology of cor pulmonale in COPD. Am J Respir Crit Care Med 1994;150(Part 2):833–852.
38. Baum GL, Schwartz A, Llamas R, et al. Left ventricular function in COLD. N Engl J Med 1971;281:361–364.
39. Jezek KV, Schrijen R. LV function in COPD with and without cardiac failure. Clin Sci Molec Med 1973;45:267–279.
40. Montes de Oca M, Rassulo J, Celli B. Relationship between O_2 pulse and intrathoracic pressure in COPD patients. Chest 1995;108:155S.

Part II

Chronic Cor Pulmonale:
A Hormonal Disease

Mark O. Farber, M.D.

The development of peripheral edema in advanced chronic obstructive pulmonary disease (COPD) is a commonly observed phenomenon often referred to as "cor pulmonale" and/or "right heart failure."[1,2] Cor pulmonale has been defined as "alteration in the structure and function of the right ventricle resulting from diseases affecting the function and/or structure of the lungs."[3] Heart failure in the usual sense, i.e., a decrease in cardiac output, is not a feature of cor pulmonale with edema; in fact, cardiac output at rest may be elevated.[2,4–7]

The "classic" view that hypoxia in COPD, which leads to pulmonary hypertension, right ventricular volume overload, systemic venous hypertension, and leakage of sodium rich fluid into the interstitial space resulting in edema, has been challenged on a number of fronts.[1,2,6] The above "mechanism" of edema formation is not usually invoked for patients with congestive heart failure (CHF) who actually have higher right-sided pressures than comparably ill patients with COPD and edema.[6,8] In fact, distinguishing between the edema of respiratory and cardiac origin may be difficult. Left ventricular dysfunction and COPD often co-exist since they share the same target population. Clinical findings such as dyspnea, orthopnea, cyanosis, and cardiomegaly with gallop sounds are common in both. Electrocardiographic evidence of right ventricular hypertrophy may be specific but lacks sensitivity. In acutely ill patients, the presence of poor peripheral perfusion (low cardiac output) and pleural fluid, i.e., increased pulmonary venous pressure may help to differentiate the two as these findings are typical for left-sided failure and are generally not seen in decompensated patients with COPD. Laboratory examinations such as arterial blood gases and echocardiograms may also help to resolve the issue.[1,6]

The pathophysiologic mechanism(s) that produce edema in COPD patients can be shown to be remarkably similar to those subtending edema formation in CHF: both are caused by similar functional renal impairments; CHF due to low cardiac output and COPD due to hypercapneic acidosis.[1,10] Specific knowledge of the pathogenic mechanisms involved in producing these derangements in sodium, water, and hormonal metabolism should provide a pathway toward more rational modalities of therapy.

As suggested by Campbell and Short[11] many years ago, the prerequisite for edema in COPD patients is the retention of carbon dioxide, which initiates a cascade of events heralded by increasing sodium retention, increased plasma norepinephrine, diminished renal blood flow, increased levels of plasma renin activity (PRA), angiotensin II (AII), and plasma aldosterone (PA).[1,12] Hyponatremia, secondary to inappropriate secretion of arginine vasopressin (AVP, antidiuretic hormone) occurs less often and may be related to baroreceptor stimulation and/or to stimulation of AVP by AII.[12–14] Edema in COPD can and does occur in the absence of significant hypoxemia, i.e., arterial pO_2 >60 torr; however, decompensated cor pulmonale with edema and hyponatremia occurs more frequently when significant hypoxemia is also present.[1] The independent role of hypoxemia in the production of the above disturbances remains unclear. Similarly, the specific role of atrial natriuretic peptide (ANP) in the above mix of physiologic derangements remains to be elucidated. Even though definite reciprocal relationships under normal physiologic conditions have been demonstrated between ANP and the PRA-PA axis, these appear to be absent in COPD and CHF patients.[15–18]

Patients with stable hypercapneic COPD, with arterial pO_2s usually <60 torr, can uniformly be shown to have a decrease in effective renal plasma flow (ERPF) and an increase in total body sodium even in the absence of peripheral edema. The level of ERPF is inversely correlated with the arterial pCO_2 level and there is a diminished capacity to excrete sodium and water in these patients, which directly correlates with the reduction in ERPF.[1,12,19] Little change can be demonstrated in the glomerular filtration rate (GFR), and the filtration fraction (FF) rises.[12]

Along with the observed changes in renal function there are hormonal perturbations. Plasma norepinephrine, an indicator of the level of renal sympathetic tone, becomes elevated early in the course of the disease as hypercapnia develops.[1,20,21] ANP is also likely to be elevated relatively early in the course of the disease before edema is evident[2,22–25] and increases further as decompensation occurs.[2,26] Attempts have been made to correlate ANP elevations in COPD with PaO_2 level, right atrial pressure, and pulmonary artery pressure[23,25,27,28] with limited success. Evidence indicates that ANP release is a function of changes in right or left atrial transmural pressures or effective filling pressures (EFP), which are both likely to be elevated in severe COPD.[24,29,30] Later in the course of COPD, but often before edema is manifest, there may be subtle increases in the PRA-AII-PA axis.[1,12,21] Eventually, 40%–50% of edematous patients with COPD will manifest evidence of secondary hyperaldosteronism with increased plasma levels of PA, AII, and PRA.[1,12,31]

Approximately 10% of edematous COPD patients are hyponatremic (plasma sodium <130 mEq/L). All of the patients with hyponatremia have inappropriately elevated levels of AVP for the corresponding level of plasma osmolality,[1,12,14,32] as well as an enhanced AVP response to infusion of hypertonic saline.[1,13]

The profile of renal function and hormonal changes in the course of COPD are summarized in Table 1. COPD patients with normocapnia and mild hypoxemia (Stage I) display normal renal and hormonal function.[33,34] Note the earlier onset of renal functional impairment and ANP elevation in Stage II (hypercapnia and moderate hypoxemia) as compared to the onset of other hormonal abnormalities later in the disease. Stage III (hypercapnia and moderate-severe hypoxemia) occurs when edema and hyponatremia are prevalent.

_____ **Table 1** _____

Profile of Renal and Hormonal Function in COPD Progression

	Stage I (Normocapnia Mild Hypoxemia)	Stage II (Hypercapnia, Moderate Hypoxemia)	Stage III (Hypercapnia, Moderate–severe Hypoxemia)
Peripheral edema	—	±	+ +*#
Hyponatremia	—	—	+*#
Glomerular filtration rate (GFR)	N	N ± ↓	↓
Effective renal plasma flow (ERPF)	N	↓ ↓*	↓ ↓ ↓*#
Filtration fraction (FF)	N	↑*	↑ ↑*#
4 hour H$_2$O excretion	N	↓ ↓*	↓ ↓ ↓*#
4 hour Na$^+$ excretion	N	↓ ↓*	↓ ↓ ↓*
Plasma norepinephrine	N	↑*	↑ ↑*#
Plasma renin activity (PRA)	N	N ± ↑	↑*#
Angiotension II (AII)	N	N ± ↑	↑*#
Plasma aldosterone (PA)	N	N ± ↑	↑*#
Atrial natriuretic peptide (ANP)	N	↑*	↑ ↑*#
Arginine vasopressin (AVP; for corresponding posm)	N	N ± ↑	↑*#

*P < 0.05 versus Stage I.
#P < 0.05 versus Stage II.
Severity indicated is the average for each stage.

Edematous patients with advanced lung disease are not in a state of "heart failure" since numerous investigations have shown normal to elevated cardiac output in such patients; in most instances both right atrial and systemic venous pressures are mildly elevated or normal.[6,20,35–39] As CO_2 retention begins, even without severe hypoxemia, renal function declines along with the cellular (and extracellular pH). The renal response is to increase the rate of tubular sodium-hydrogen exchange increasing bicarbonate reabsorption over the entire nephron.[40] Thus, there is a net increase in sodium reabsorption as bicarbonate excretion is minimized. Sympathetic tone is enhanced likely due to the intracellular acidosis and an increase in the plasma level of norepinephrine is seen.[20,21] Enhanced renal sympathetic tone diminishes ERPF, further increasing tubular sodium reabsorption and may also promote a redistribution in renal blood flow.[41] Since GFR remains relatively stable FF increases, causing a rise in peritubular oncotic pressure inducing even more tubular sodium reabsorption.[1] Patients with COPD, hypercapnia, and mild hypoxemia, therefore, cannot normally excrete a sodium or water load.[12,33,34] As renal perfusion declines, perhaps due to a decrease in arterial blood volume or "effective circulating volume,"[10] additional stimulation of the PRA-AII-PA axis often occurs, which further exacerbates renal sodium retention. The declining ability to excrete sodium along with the progressive diminution in renal perfusion, possibly aggravated by worsening hypoxemia, invariably leads to edema formation.[1,2]

It would appear almost axiomatic that ANP would rise to offset the propensity toward sodium retention evoked by low renal perfusion and high aldosterone secretion. ANPs structure and, to some extent, its function, have been described.[42] Its release from both atria is stimulated by small (1–2 mmHg) increases in atrial pressure, at least in animal studies.[42] In normals, it promotes natriuresis and diuresis, lowers PRA and PA, and inhibits AVP release.[43–45] ANP has been shown to be elevated in advanced COPD increasing as the disease progresses.[2,18,22,26] Levels observed in COPD are generally lower than those seen in patients with left-sided CHF[43,45,46] and consistently higher than in subjects with liver cirrhosis.[47]

The precise role of ANP in the congestive state of COPD remains to be elucidated. Studies[1,15] suggest that the normal suppressing effect of ANP on aldosterone is not demonstrable in edematous COPD patients, perhaps because this suppressing potential is overridden by the stimulatory effect of decreased renal perfusion on the PRA-PA axis; it has been noted that the increased level of ANP does not prevent sodium and water retention in COPD patients.[18] It may be that in COPD patients, as proposed for patients with CHF, the primary function of the ANP system is in acute states, where it contributes to unloading the central venous, right heart, and pulmonary blood volumes.[17,18] Conversely, the primary function of the PRA-AII-PA axis, is in chronic conditions, where it contributes to the support of the arterial volume.[48] This concept is supported by the observation that ANP is elevated in COPD prior to the stimulation of the renin-aldosterone axis. A comparison of patients with COPD versus those with CHF can be found in Table 2.

Theoretically, transmural right and/or left atrial pressure changes should be the primary stimuli for release of ANP.[44] Transmural pressure can also be defined as effective filling pressure (EFP), the difference between atrial pressure and intrathoracic or intrapleural pressure. Measurements of EFP in both patients with CHF and COPD as it affects ANP release are few. Patients with CHF have both high left and right atrial pressures with intrathoracic pressures presumably close to normal; therefore, EFP will be significantly elevated.

The situation regarding right-sided cardiac and pleural pressures in COPD may not be as obvious. Contrary to "clinical intuition" breathing at high lung volumes, as with severe COPD, leads to large negative pleural pressure swings during inspiration and minimal elevation during expiration. Thus the mean pleural pressure in advanced COPD or in exacerbations of COPD and/or asthma should be significantly negative.[39,49] Right

___ **Table 2** _____

Edematous COPD Patients versus Edematous Cardiac Patients

	CHF	COPD
Hemodynamics		
Heart rate	↑	↑
Cardiac output	↓	N ± ↑
Pulmonary artery pressure	±↑	↑↑
Pulmonary artery wedge pressure	↑↑↑	N ± ↑
Right ventricular end-diastolic pressure	↑	N ± ↑
Right atrial pressure	↑↑	N ± ↑
Right atrial transmural pressure	↑	↑
Left atrial transmural pressure	↑↑↑	↑
Respiratory Dynamics		
Intrathoracic (pleural) pressure (mean)	N	N ± ↑
Renal Function		
Glomerular filtration rate (GFR)	N ± ↓	N ± ↓
Effective renal plasma flow (ERPF)	↓↓	↓↓
Filtration fraction (FF)	↑	↑
4-hour H_2O excretion	↓	↓
4-hour Na^+ excretion	↓	↓
Hormonal Function		
Plasma renin activity (PRA)	↑↑	↑
Angiotensin II (AII)	↑↑	↑
Plasma aldosterone (PA)	↑↑	↑
Atrial natriuretic peptide (ANP)	↑↑↑	↑↑
Arginine vasopressin (AVP; for corresponding Posm)	↑	↑

Severity indicated is the average for each group.

atrial pressure in severe COPD again, perhaps surprisingly, may be normal or only mildly elevated.[6,23,50–52] Perhaps the negative pleural pressure prevents right atrial pressure from rising even in the face of hypoxemia. Indeed, positive correlations can be demonstrated between intrathoracic pressure and left atrial pressure as assessed by pulmonary capillary wedge pressure in COPD patients.[53] The effects of intrathoracic pressure changes on right atrial pressure in hypoxemic COPD patients were not recorded. In any event, it seems that the net result in severe COPD is that right atrial EFP will increase as pleural pressure becomes more negative and right atrial pressure either remains normal or increases. Interestingly, left atrial EFP in patients with COPD has been shown to be elevated with intrathoracic pressures largely negative especially in patients with advanced COPD and hypercapnia.[29] Measurements of right atrial EFP in advanced COPD patients are not available or were made only at end-expiration[22] underscoring the still many unanswered questions concerning pulmonary hemodynamics in COPD.[54]

Supporting data for the above conceptual framework may be gleaned from the literature. In normals, changes in EFP have been shown to be the controlling factor for ANP release; even when atrial volume is decreasing, ANP increases as a function of enhanced right atrial EFP produced by positive pressure breathing in normals.[30] In mechanically ventilated patients without significant heart or lung disease, changes in ANP were shown to be directly correlated with changes in EFP.[55,56] ANP elevations in COPD seem to correlate with the degree of lung disease present as assessed by the presence of hypercapnia or by the magnitude of pulmonary hypertension.[2,25,57] According to the above scheme, hypercapneic patients would have the greatest degree of airway obstruction, the greatest degree of hypoxemia, the greatest discrepancy between intrathoracic and right atrial pressure and, therefore, the greatest increase in right atrial EFP and, therefore, the greatest increases in ANP. The above conceptual frame can also explain the acute antidiuresis seen with nasal CPAP (continuous positive airway pressure) in patients with obstructive sleep apnea[58,59]; CPAP (PEEP, positive end-expiratory pressure) eliminates the large negative pleural pressure swings generated by upper airway obstruction resulting in decreased EFP and suppression of ANP.

Exercise may cause further increases in ANP in normals and in COPD patients.[16,23,57,60] Presumably, pleural pressure remains negative or decreases further while right atrial pressure increases resulting in an increase in EFP. The above hypotheses can be easily tested.

The mechanisms subtending the inappropriate release of AVP in advanced COPD most likely involve non-osmotic stimuli. AII may stimulate AVP directly, but this notion is debated.[61] Some support for this concept comes from a clinical study[13] where administration of an angiotensin converting enzyme (ACE) inhibitor normalized the slope of the AVP/Posm line in hypercapneic COPD, implying that a reduction in AII was responsible. As mentioned above, hypercapneic COPD with edema may be associated with a decreased arterial blood volume, much like decompensated cirrhosis and CHF. The effective low circulating volume in addition to stimulating PRA, AII, and PA also results in baroreceptor firing and in the non-osmotic release of AVP.[10,61] Measurements of "effective circulating volume" in edematous COPD patients, defined as the discrepancy between the circulating arterial blood volume and the vascular capacity of the circulation, have not been published.

It is clear that hyponatremia in COPD patients is always associated with "inappropriate" antidiuretic hormone secretion,[12,14,32] since these patients have plasma AVP levels inappropriately high for plasma osmolality even if plasma sodium levels fall within the normal range. It is recognized that in patients with inappropriate AVP secretion, plasma sodium may be normal unless water intake is excessive.[1,7,12]

Dopamine has been putatively invoked in the pathogenesis of edema formation in COPD. Dopamine receptors in the renal tubules and vasculature when stimulated promote sodium excretion, renal vasodilation, and an increase in GFR. Dopamine also can inhibit renin release. Preliminary studies in COPD patients demonstrate increased urinary dopamine excretion in those patients with respiratory failure and edema, which fall during convalescence. Renal dopamine output correlated with the degree of hypercapnia.[2] Further studies are clearly needed to clarify the role of dopamine in the pathogenesis of the sodium and water abnormalities of COPD.

Another "hormone," brain natriuretic peptide (BNP), a substance first isolated from porcine brains has properties similar to those of ANP. BNP is elaborated predominantly by the cardiac ventricles and has been found to be elevated in patients with CHF[62,63] as well as in COPD patients.[64] BNP levels in COPD correlated with the degree of hypoxemia and were proportionately higher than ANP levels in the same patients. To date, only one study of elevated BNP in COPD has been published.[64] Further work is needed to establish any relationship between BNP and ANP in the congestive state of COPD and whether one or the other is predominant.

Another natriuretic peptide, C-type natriuretic peptide (CNP), which is synthesized by vascular endothelium, has been found to be elevated in patients with severe COPD but not in patients with CHF. In dogs, CNP, contrary to the actions of ANP and BNP caused profound hypotension and reduced cardiac output and decreased sodium excretion, i.e., antinatriuretic.[65]

The independent role of hypoxemia in the pathogenesis of sodium and water retention in COPD remains open. Removal of supplemental oxygen in hypercapneic COPD subjects, resulting in acute hypoxemia, diminished patients' ability to excrete a sodium load, while acute hypoxemia of similar degree in normocapneic individuals had no measurable effect.[21] Longer-term studies in hypoxemic, hypercapneic COPD patients consisting of 1 week of oxygen supplementation resulted in significant natriuresis.[66] Further, in edematous patients with acute respiratory failure secondary to COPD, diuresis resulted from oxygen therapy except when PRA and PA were extremely high.[4] Animal studies lend support to these clinical investigations.[67] Hormonal changes resulting from O$_2$ removal have generally shown no significant change in hormonal parameters including AVP.[21,22,31,65] On balance, hypoxemia can be inferred to worsen the renal and hormonal effects of hypercapnia.

Therapies that are often applied to COPD patients may exacerbate already existing problems such as hypochloremia and tachyarrhythmias. Relatively little use of ACE inhibitors has been reported in COPD patients.

These drugs, at least in patients with CHF, enhance sodium excretion by blocking the generation of AII and PA, while ERPF is increased.[10] In an acute study in COPD patients, ACE inhibition has been shown to be natriuretic through a diminution in renal tubular sodium reabsorption at constant ERPF while it normalized the AVP/Posm relationship.[13] However, another acute study in COPD patients found no positive effect of ACE inhibition on sodium excretion.[68] In a more prolonged trial, 1 month of ACE inhibition in hypoxic COPD patients significantly improved ERPF.[69] Although it may seem logical that ACE inhibitors should be used with or without oxygen administration to treat edematous COPD patients, further clinical studies are needed in order to establish the efficacy of this approach.

An overview of the pathogenesis of sodium and water metabolism in COPD is depicted in Figure 1. Solid arrows indicate relatively well established pathways/mechanisms, broken arrows indicate pathways/mechanisms postulated or not well established. The linchpin in this scheme is an

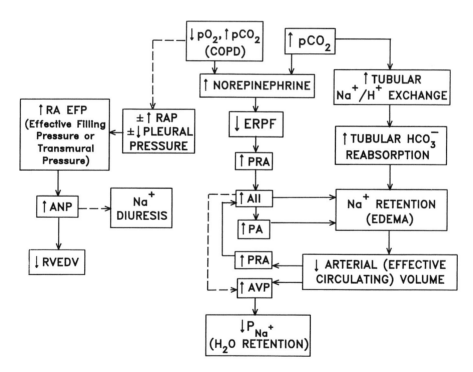

Figure 1. For description see text. AII - angiotensin II; ANP = atrial natriuretic peptide; AVP = arginine vasopressin (antidiuretic hormone); ERPF = effective renal plasma flow; PA = plasma aldosterone; PRA = plasma renin activity; RAP = right atrial pressure; RVEDV = right ventricular end-diastolic volume.

elevation in the pCO_2 that initiates a cascade of events and reactions, almost entirely due to the induced intracellular and extracellular acidosis. The compensatory changes tending to correct the respiratory acidosis lead to increased renal sodium reabsorption, catecholamine secretion, and diminished effective renal plasma flow. The resultant renal hypoperfusion secondary to low renal blood flow and low arterial volume eventually effects a state of secondary hyperaldosteronism with increased PRA, AII, and PA, which worsens the sodium retention. Reflex baroreceptor activation caused by the low volume state stimulates AVP secretion priming the patient for the development of hyponatremia.

On the left of Figure 1, severe COPD as indicated by CO_2 retention and hypoxemia may cause the mean intrathoracic pressure to decline (large negative inspiratory swings with expiratory swings only minimally increased) as right atrial pressure either increases or remains normal. The net result is often an increase in right atrial filling or transmural pressure/effective filling pressure—the difference between right atrial pressure and intrathoracic or intrapleural pressure. An increase in EFP is the primary stimulus for atrial release of ANP, which directly antagonizes cardiac pressure and volume overload. Whether the level of ANP observed in congested states promotes a tendency toward a sodium diuresis remains an open question. Left atrial EFP also tends to be elevated in COPD patients and may also contribute to ANP release.

References

1. Farber MO, Manfredi F. Sodium and water metabolism in COPD. In: Cherniack NS (ed). Chronic Obstructive Pulmonary Disease. Philadelphia, W.B. Saunders Co., 1991, pp. 216–221.
2. MacNee W. Pathophysiology of cor pulmonale in chronic obstructive pulmonary disease. Part II. Am J Respir Crit Care Med 1994;150:1158–1168.
3. Behnke RH, Blount SG, Bristol W, et al. Primary prevention of pulmonary heart disease. Circulation 1970;41:A17–A23.
4. Leading article. Oedema in cor pulmonale. Lancet 1975;2:1289–1290.
5. MacNee W. Right ventricular function in cor pulmonale. Cardiology 1988; 75(Suppl 1):30–40.
6. MacNee W. Pathophysiology of cor pulmonale in chronic obstructive pulmonary disease. Part I. Am J Respir Crit Care Med 1994;150:833–852.
7. Richens JM, Howard P. Oedema in cor pulmonale. Clin Sci 1982;62:255–259.
8. Guazzi MD, Agostoni P, Perego B, et al. Apparent paradox of neurohumoral axis inhibition after body fluid volume depletion in patients with chronic congestive heart failure and water retention. Br Heart J 1994;72:534–539.
9. Packer M. Neurohormonal interactions and adaptations in congestive heart failure. Circulation 1988;77(4):721–730.
10. Schrier RW. Body fluid volume regulation in health and disease: A unifying hypothesis. Ann Intern Med 1990;113:155–159.

11. Campbell EJM, Short DS. The cause of oedema in "cor pulmonale". Lancet 1960;i:1184–1186.
12. Farber MO, Roberts LR, Weinberger MH, et al. Abnormalities of sodium and H_2O handling in chronic obstructive lung disease. Arch Intern Med 1982;142:1326–1330.
13. Farber MO, Weinberger MH, Robertson GL, et al. The effects of angiotensin converting enzyme inhibition on sodium handling in patients with advanced chronic obstructive lung disease. Am Rev Respir Dis 1987;136:862–866.
14. Farber MO, Weinberger MH, Robertson GL, et al. Hormonal abnormalities affecting sodium and water balance in acute respiratory failure due to chronic obstructive lung disease. Chest 1984;85:49–54.
15. Carlone S, Palange P, Mannix ET, et al. Atrial natriuretic peptide, renin and aldosterone in obstructive lung disease and heart failure. Am J Med Sci 1989;298(4):243–248.
16. Mannix ET, Manfredi F, Palange P, et al. The effect of O_2 with exercise on atrial natriuretic peptide in chronic obstructive lung disease. Chest 1992;101:341–344.
17. Rogers TK, Sheedy W, Waterhouse J, et al. Haemodynamic effects of atrial natriuretic peptide in hypoxic chronic obstructive pulmonary disease. Thorax 1994;49:233–239.
18. Skwarski K, Lee M, Turnbull L, et al. Atrial natriuretic peptide in stable and decompensated chronic obstructive pulmonary disease. Thorax 1993;48:730–735.
19. Bauer FK, Telfer N, Herbst HH, et al. Hyponatremia and increased exchangeable sodium in chronic obstructive lung disease. Am J Med Sci 1965;250:245–253.
20. Henriksen JH, Christensen NJ, Kok-Jensen A, et al. Increased plasma noradrenaline concentration in patients with chronic obstructive lung disease: Relation to haemodynamics and blood gases. Scand J Clin Lab Invest 1980;40:419–427.
21. Reihman DA, Farber MO, Weinberger MH, et al. Effect of hypoxemia on sodium and water excretion in chronic obstructive lung disease. Am J Med 1985;78:87–94.
22. Adnot S, Andrivet P, Chabrier P, et al. Plasma levels of atrial natriuretic factor, renin activity, and aldosterone in patients with chronic obstructive pulmonary disease. Response to O_2 removal and to hyperoxia. Am Rev Respir Dis 1990;141:1178–1184.
23. Adnot S, Chabrier PE, Andrivet P, et al. Atrial natriuretic peptide concentrations and pulmonary hemodynamics in patients with pulmonary artery hypertension. Am Rev Respir Dis 1987;136:951–956.
24. Adnot S, Sediame S, Defouilloy C, et al. Role of atrial natriuretic factor in impaired sodium excretion of normocapnic and hypercapnic patients with chronic obstructive lung disease. Am Rev Respir Dis 1993;148:1049–1055.
25. Burghuber OC, Hartter E, Punzengruber CH, et al. Human atrial natriuretic peptide secretion in precapillary pulmonary hypertension. Clinical study in patients with COPD and interstitial fibrosis. Chest 1988;93:31–37.
26. Neilly JB, Doyle J, Stevenson RD. Atrial natriuretic peptide levels in decompensated and treated cor pulmonale. (abstract) Am Rev Respir Dis 1988;137(Part 2):187.
27. Davidson AC, Winter RJD, Treacher DF, et al. Increased atrial natriuretic factor in chronically hypoxaemic patients with pulmonary hypertension. Am Rev Respir Dis 1988;137(Suppl, 4 Part 2):105.
28. Winter RJD, Davidson AC, Treacher D, et al. Atrial natriuretic peptide concentrations in hypoxic secondary pulmonary hypertension: Relation to haemody-

namic and blood gas variables and response to supplemental oxygen. Thorax 1989;44:58–62.

29. Albert RK, Muramoto A, Caldwell J, et al. Increases in intrathoracic pressure do not explain the rise in left ventricular end-diastolic pressure that occurs during exercise in patients with chronic obstructive pulmonary disease. Am Rev Respir Dis 1985;132:623–627.

30. Mannix ET, Farber MO, Aronoff GR, et al. Regulation of atrial natriuretic peptide release in normal humans. J Appl Physiol 1991;71(4):1340–1345.

31. Raff H, Levy SA. Renin-angiotensin II-aldosterone and ACTH-cortisol control during acute hypoxemia and exercise in patients with chronic obstructive pulmonary disease. Am Rev Respir Dis 1986;133:396–399.

32. Szatalowicz VL, Goldberg JP, Anderson RJ. Plasma antidiuretic hormone in acute respiratory failure. Am J Med 1982;72:583–587.

33. Farber MO, Bright TP, Strawbridge RA, et al. Impaired water handling in chronic obstructive lung disease. J Lab Clin Med 1975;85:41–49.

34. Farber MO, Kiblawi SO, Strawbridge RA, et al. Studies of plasma vasopressin and the renin-angiotensin-aldosterone system in chronic obstructive lung disease. J Lab Clin Med 1977;90:373–380.

35. Dexter L, Whittenberger JL, Gorlin R, et al. The effect of chronic pulmonary disease (cor pulmonale and hypoxia) on the dynamics of the circulation in man. Trans Assoc Am Physicians 1951;64:226–236.

36. Harvey RM, Ferrer MI, Richards DW Jr, et al. Influence of chronic pulmonary disease on the heart and circulation. Am J Med 1951;10:719–738.

37. Mounsey JPD, Ritzmann LW, Selverstone NJ, et al. Circulatory changes in severe pulmonary emphysema. Br Heart J 1952;14:153–172.

38. Robertson GL. Diseases of the posterior pituitary. In: Felig P, Baxter J, Broadus AE, et al. (eds). Endocrinology and Metabolism. New York, McGraw-Hill Book Co., 1981, pp. 251–277.

39. Wise RA. COPD and the peripheral circulation. In: Cherniack NS (ed). Chronic Obstructive Pulmonary Disease. Philadelphia, PA, WB Saunders Co., 1991, pp. 167–177.

40. Molony DA, Jacobson HR. Respiratory acid-base disorders. In: Kokko JP, Tannen RL (eds). Fluids and Electrolytes. Philadelphia, PA, WB Saunders Company, 1986, pp. 305–381.

41. DiBona GF. Catecholamines and neuroadrenergic control of renal function. In: Dunn MJ (ed). Renal Endocrinology. Baltimore, MD, Williams & Wilkins, 1983, pp. 323–366.

42. Needleman P, Adams SP, Cole BR, et al. Atriopeptins as cardiac hormones. Hypertension 1985;7(4):469–482.

43. Raine AEG, Erne P, Burgisser E, et al. Atrial natriuretic peptide and atrial pressure in patients with congestive heart failure. N Engl J Med 1986;315(9): 533–537.

44. Palluk R, Gaida W, Hoefke W. Minireview. Atrial natriuretic factor. Life Sci 1985;36(15):1415–1425.

45. Shenker Y, Sider RS, Ostafin EA, et al. Plasma levels of immunoreactive atrial natriuretic factor in healthy subjects and in patients with edema. J Clin Invest 1985;76:1684–1687.

46. Burnett JC Jr, Kao PC, Hu DC, et al. Atrial natriuretic peptide elevation in congestive heart failure in the human. Science 1986;231:1145–1147.

47. Gerbes AL, Arendt RM, Ritter D, et al. Plasma atrial natriuretic factor in patients with cirrhosis. N Engl J Med 1985;313(25):1609–1610.

48. Laragh JH. The endocrine control of blood volume, blood pressure and sodium balance: Atrial hormone and renin system—interactions. J Hypertens 1986; 4(Suppl 2):S143–S156.

49. Kitchin AH, Lowther CP, Matthews MB. The effects of exercise and of breathing oxygen-enriched air on the pulmonary circulation in emphysema. Clin Sci 1961;21:93–106.

50. Andrivet P, Chabrier P, Defouilloy C, et al. Intravenously administered atrial natriuretic factor in patients with COPD. Effects on ventilation-perfusion relationships and pulmonary hemodynamics. Chest 1994;106:118–124.

51. Harris P, Segel N, Green I, et al. The influence of the airways resistance and alveolar pressure on the pulmonary vascular resistance in chronic bronchitis. Cardiovasc Res 1968;2:84–92.

52. Segel N, Bishop JM. The circulation in patients with chronic bronchitis and emphysema at rest and during exercise, with special reference to the influence of changes in blood viscosity and blood volume on the pulmonary circulation. J Clin Invest 1966;45(10):1555–1568.

53. Lim TPK, Brownlee WE. Pulmonary hemodynamics in obstructive lung disease. Dis Chest 1968;53(2):113–125.

54. Butler J. The heart is not always in good hands. Chest 1990;97(2):453–460.

55. Andrivet P, Adnot S, Brun-Buisson C, et al. Involvement of ANF in the acute antidiuresis during PEEP ventilation. J Appl Physiol 1988;65(5):1967–1974.

56. Andrivet P, Adnot S, Sanker S, et al. Hormonal interactions and renal function during mechanical ventilation and ANF infusion in humans. J Appl Physiol 1991;70(1):287–292.

57. Graudal N, Gallòe AM, Storm T, et al. Atrial natriuretic peptide (ANP) in chronic obstructive pulmonary disease (COPD): The relationship between plasma ANP and lung function. Effects of exercise and of the calcium antagonist, isradipine, on plasma ANP. A randomized, double-blind, placebo-controlled study. Horm Metab Res 1992;24:130–133.

58. Baruzzi A, Riva R, Cirignotta F, et al. Atrial natriuretic peptide and catecholamines in obstructive sleep apnea syndrome. Sleep 1991;14(1):83–86.

59. Rodenstein RO, D'Odemont JP, Pieters T, et al. Diurnal and nocturnal diuresis and natriuresis in obstructive sleep apnea. Effects of nasal continuous positive airway pressure therapy. Am Rev Respir Dis 1992;145(6):1367–1371.

60. Mannix ET, Palange P, Aronoff GR, et al. Atrial natriuretic peptide and the renin-aldosterone axis during exercise in man. Med Sci Sports Exerc 1990; 22(6):785–789.

61. Schrier RW, Bichet DG. Osmotic and nonosmotic control of vasopressin release and the pathogenesis of impaired water excretion in adrenal, thyroid, and edematous disorders. J Lab Clin Med 1981;98(1):1–15.

62. Florkowski CM, Richards AM, Espiner EA, et al. Renal, endocrine, and hemodynamic interactions of atrial and brain natriuretic peptides in normal men. Am J Physiol 1994;266(4 Part 2):R1244–R1250.

63. Hill NS, Klinger JR, Warburton RR, et al. Brain natriuretic peptide: Possible role in the modulation of hypoxic pulmonary hypertension. Am J Physiol 1994;266: L308–L315.

64. Lang CC, Coutie WJ, Struthers AD, et al. Elevated levels of brain natriuretic peptide in acute hypoxaemic chronic obstructive pulmonary disease. Clin Sci 1992;83:529–533.

65. Cargill RI, Barr CS, Coutie WJ, et al. C-type natriuretic peptide levels in cor pulmonale and in congestive heart failure. Thorax 1994;49:1247–1249.

66. Mannix ET, Dowdeswell IRG, Carlone S, et al. The effect of oxygen on sodium excretion in hypoxemic patients with chronic obstructive lung disease. Chest 1990;97:840–844.
67. Rose CE Jr, Kimmel DP, Godine RL Jr, et al. Synergistic effects of acute hypoxemia and hypercapnic acidosis in conscious dogs. Renal dysfunction and activation of the renin-angiotensin system. Circ Res 1983;53:202–213.
68. Stewart AG, Waterhouse JC, Billings CG, et al. Effects of angiotensin converting enzyme inhibition on sodium excretion in patients with hypoxaemic chronic obstructive pulmonary disease. Thorax 1994;49(10):995–998.
69. Oliver RM, Peacock AJ, Fleming JS, et al. Renal and pulmonary effects of angiotensin converting enzyme inhibition in chronic hypoxic lung disease. Thorax 1989;44:513–515.

Chapter 8

Mechanical Ventilation

Anthony M. Cosentino, M.D.

Mechanical Ventilation

Eschew obfuscation. A ventilator is simply a force generator that when applied to a subject's airway is capable of generating a flow of gas into the lungs. As occurs in spontaneous ventilation, exhalation is passive. The source of energy may be electrical, pneumatic, or mechanical. Gas flow may be initiated by a program within the apparatus and/or by the subject's effort. The simplest of ventilators is an anesthesia bag that is manually powered by the operator's hand(s) at a rate that is deemed to be appropriate for the patient, a topic of significant complexity, which will be treated in the section on ventilator strategies.

Ventilators were once designated as being volume ventilators or pressure ventilators. This terminology has little to be said for it since all ventilation is the result of a positive pressure gradient and the goal is the delivery of an adequate volume of gas at a reasonable frequency. However, there is a lesson to be learned. The pressure versus volume ventilator controversy took place in the 1960s and in fact referred to what mechanical settings the technician (therapist, nurse, physician) made on the face panel and it was generally assumed that these settings referred to what terminated the inspiratory phase. A Bird Mark VII (Bird Product Co., Palm Springs, CA, USA) required that a pressure be set and inspiration was terminated when the preset pressure was attained at the ambient port and thus it was referred to as pressure cycled. The Bennett PR I and PR II (Nellcor Puritan Bennett, Carlsbad, CA, USA)

From: Cosentino AM, Martin RJ (eds.): Cardiothoracic Interrelationships in Clinical Practice. © Futura Publishing Co., Inc., Armonk, NY, 1996.

also required setting a pressure, however, this was a systems pressure that was present when the valve opened at the onset of inspiration. Inspiration terminated when the flow rate across the valve fell to 1/4 L/sec. The valve was flow sensitive, not unlike some of today's pressure support circuitry (see pressure support ventilation [PSV]), which has been variously designated as pressure-limited or pressure-preset ventilation (Figure 1).

In the 1960s there was an awareness that what in fact we sought was a volume of ventilation and that pressure was a means to an end and so volume ventilators were "rediscovered." Volume ventilators, Morch and Engstrom, actually preceded the generation of pressure cycled ventilators. An early model of the recent genre was the Emerson (J.H. Emerson Co., Cambridge, MA, USA). This in fact was and is a time cycled ventilator, inspiratory and expiratory times are electrically set and a preset volume is delivered from a cylinder. This machine was and still is a work horse. Unfortunately the original model, which was ideal for a paralyzed patient, lacked the flexibility to respond to a non-paralyzed patient's efforts for an additional breath or two. There was the potential for development of the dysphasic patient-ventilator interface and consequent risk of barotrauma.

The "pressure" models had the advantage that they could respond to a patient's inspiratory efforts and at least theoretically should minimize asynchronous ventilation. Unfortunately, resistances in the circuitry often went unrecognized, as in the Bennett Cascade humidifier, and asynchrony often

Constant Pressure Ventilation 40 cm H₂O*

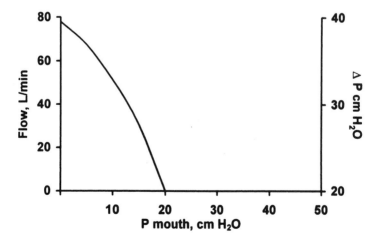

Figure 1. Note pressure-controlled ventilation and Bennett PR II, "pressure cycled" ventilator patterns are identical. Ventilator turns off at a flow rate near 0, i.e., 1/4 L/sec and $\Delta P > 0$ (flow-sensitive system).

resulted. A small aperture about 2 or 3 mm was necessary to keep moisture from getting back to the valve and disturbing its very sensitive rotary mechanism. It was through this aperture that patient effort was transmitted to the valve. With the introduction of the Bennett, MAI, volume ventilator this was no longer necessary because the valve was of a different design. Nevertheless, this construction of the humidifier persisted and remained a source of significant resistance to patient efforts to initiate ventilation.

There was no reason that pressure ventilators could not be operated to deliver a specific tidal volume (VT) at a set rate and in fact ventilator orders in our unit included a VT, respiratory frequency (f), and variable ratio (I:E). This required continuous surveillance of VT, usually with a volume displacement spirometer, and a diligent team to vary pressure as needed. This entire apparatus (Bennett PR II, humidifier, and spirometer) cost less than $1000. The peak operating pressure was 40-cm H_2O and was delivered as a square wave (see Pressure Controlled Ventilation).

Unfortunately the halcyon days of the 1960s continued into the 1970s. Hospitals were paid their charges and medicine clamored for bells and whistles. Why should a therapist and/or nurse have to watch a VT and re-set a ventilator every couple of hours when a machine could do this and free the therapist to give needless intermittent positive pressure breathing treatments? And so volume ventilators became de rigueur and unlike the first generation they could respond to patients' inspiratory efforts and deliver a preset volume and so we had a ventilator capable of behaving in an assist-control mode. I prefer to call this volume assist-control as contrasted with the pressure cycled ventilators, which functioned as pressure assist-control.

About this time, Ashbaugh et al.[1] reported that increasing end-expiratory pressures above atmospheric could decrease pulmonary arterio-venous admixture (PA to PV) in cases of diffuse lung injury and positive end-expiratory pressure (PEEP) became a part of the lexicon. The earliest PEEP devices were spring loaded with variable tension and imposed a significant resistance to expiration.[2–4] The exception was the water column PEEP mechanism added to the Emerson ventilator. About this time, Kirby, Downs and Civetta et al.,[5] wished to use high levels of PEEP, 15–25 cm H_2O, to decrease shunt in patients, often post-op, who otherwise had good respiratory mechanics. It was reasoned they should be allowed to breath spontaneously to offset the effects of PEEP on venous return and cardiac output. The equipment they chose was an Emerson ventilator with a low resistance parallel circuit for spontaneous breathing from a pressurized anesthesia bag (Figure 2). Most breaths were to be patient initiated. This was the initial circuitry for what became known as intermittent mandatory ventilation (IMV), an unfortunate term since it stressed what the system had in common with all other ventilator strategies, i.e., intermittent machine generated breaths. What was unique was the fact that patients could choose to freely take unassisted breaths and

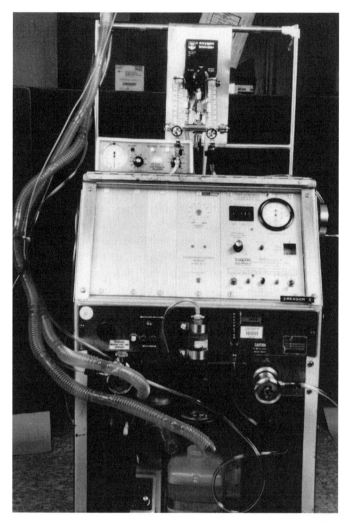

Figure 2. Mechanical ventilation. Emerson ventilator as modified by Downs and Civetta to permit spontaneous, unassisted patient breaths.

through a low resistance circuit.[5,6] The idea of super PEEP as a device for isolated instances of pulmonary shunting was short lived, but IMV soon became touted as a weaning mode. Further, it was reasoned that the machine breaths should be synchronized so as to minimize patient-ventilator asynchrony. Siemens (Siemens Medical Inc., Danvers, MA, USA) developed a ventilator, cost in excess of $20,000, with synchronized IMV. Unfortunately the effort required to activate the valve and produce adequate flow of gas through a 5-mm slit (Figures 3A and 3B) was for many patients excessive and often resulted in

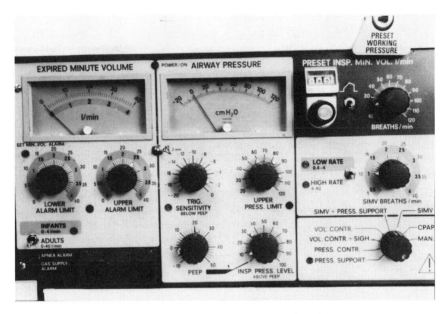

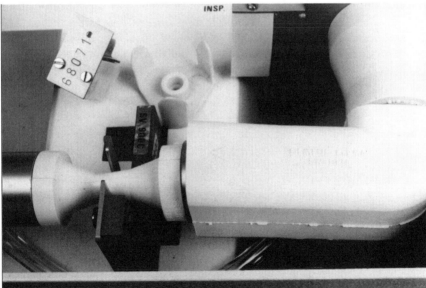

Figure 3A and 3B. Mechanical ventilation. Siemens ventilator. Note inspiratory valve includes a 5-mm slit.

very low intrapleural pressure[7–10] with significant potential for cardiovascular compromise.

MacIntyre[11] reasoned that much of this effort could be minimized by adding pressure support to the patient initiated breaths. Not surprisingly, subjects breathing through this circuitry found it to be more comfortable than IMV without pressure supported patient breaths. It is instructive to review the original paper and to note that the pressures required in this mode were about the same as those required for the machine initiated breaths. This mode is a hybrid that incorporates volume preset machine breaths with pressure supported patient initiated breaths. IMV with pressure support was originally recommended for weaning only and not as a primary ventilator mode, but who was to say when weaning should begin? Nevertheless, this is referred to as IMV with pressure support (see Weaning) and has become very popular with respiratory therapists, nurses, and physicians. It is "operator friendly." Whether it is "patient friendly" will be further examined in the section on weaning. Note that this mode per se does not decrease the patient effort to initiate a breath but rather functions to share the work of breathing once airflow has been initiated. Newer ventilator models have varied the valve mechanism to provide continuous flow in the IMV mode with a significant decrease in patient effort to initiate inspiration.[10]

An additional mode available on newer ventilators is continuous positive airways pressure (CPAP). Its use has become popular in weaning trials but frequently is imperfectly understood. For all practical purposes it is not an inspiratory assist, though there are some theoretical arguments to the contrary. However, at the onset of inspiration the open airways sense the same end-expiratory pressure and thus there is no gradient for airflow until airways pressure drops below the level of applied CPAP. This is accomplished solely by the patient's effort. Why then, should this mode have become so popular as a weaning device?

The answer lies in an understanding of auto-PEEP or intrinsic PEEP, a concept well described and popularized by Pepe and Marini (Figure 4).[12] In patients with airflow limitation, i.e., asthma and/or emphysema, it is now recognized that alveolar pressure at end-expiration may not drop to atmospheric, i.e., alveolar pressure is supra-atmospheric. The cardiovascular consequences of this phenomenon are well described in Chapter 6 and illustrated in Figure 5. In addition to the barotrauma and cardiovascular compromise that may be associated with this phenomenon there results an increase in the patient effort required to initiate airflow. Pleural pressure must decrease by an amount slightly in excess of the intrinsic PEEP (Figure 6).

It is reasoned that the addition of an equal or lesser amount of PEEP at the upper airway will result in onset of flow at airways pressure in excess of atmospheric and thus with less effort. This has in fact been shown ex-

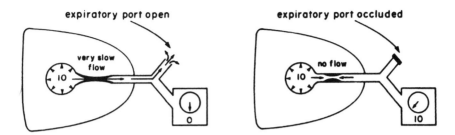

Figure 4. Mechanical ventilation. Intrinsic PEEP, detection.

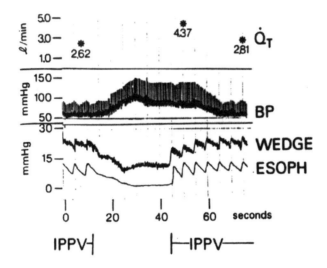

Figure 5. Mechanical ventilation. Intrinsic PEEP, cardiovascular consequences. Note that when mechanical ventilation is discontinued, esophageal pressure falls to zero, blood pressure and cardiac output increase. (Reprinted with permission from Ref. 12.)

perimentally by Smith and Marini.[13] Implied in this strategy is that the addition of PEEP does not exceed the auto-PEEP and in fact is not additive to intrinsic PEEP. In pharmacologically paralyzed patients, Tuxen[14] has reported profound cardiovascular compromise as a result of adding PEEP to paralyzed patients with asthma undergoing mechanical ventilation. Clinical experience in the non-paralyzed patient would suggest these unfavorable consequences do not occur and in fact may diminish effort required to initiate inspiration.[15] One caveat, however, not all CPAP circuitry is created equal. Continuous flow CPAP clearly requires less patient inspiratory effort[16] than non-continuous flow CPAP. Whether this is desirable during a weaning trial will be addressed in the section "Weaning."

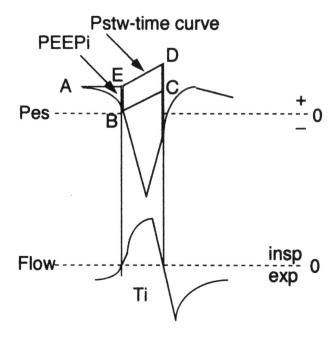

Figure 6. PTP is the sum of areas ABEA, BCDEB, and the shaded area of the Pes tracing. ED is the PSTW-time curve = $(\Delta VT/Cstw)/\Delta Ti$. EB is the degree of PEEPi. Area ABEA plus BCDEB is the portion of PTP due to PEEPi, with ABEA developed during isometric contraction of the inspiratory muscles.

In an effort to control peak pressures, a "pressure controlled" or "pressure-preset" mode has been introduced.[17,18] While peak flows and plateau pressures will be limited, mean pressure may, in fact, be greater. Appreciate that mean pressure may be an elusive value in the management of the non-paralyzed patient. The mean pressure with which we are concerned is the transpulmonary mean pressure, i.e., alveolar pressure minus pleural pressure. The latter value may be significant during patient triggered ventilation. The Consensus Conference on Mechanical Ventilation concluded that plateau pressure should be limited to 35-cm H_2O.[19] Since mean pressure is a difficult value to acquire, we can see the wisdom of their decision to look at plateau pressure. This is not to say that mean pressure is not of equal, or of greater significance, to the lung and heart. Note that during patient triggered breathing, even peak pressure is not limited in this mode, since, again, it is "translung" pressure that we must examine, i.e., mouth pressure minus pleural pressure. Pressure controlled ventilation limits the peak ventilator pressure and plateau pressure. However, in my experience, patients often appear more comfortable in this mode than in more traditional assist-control modes. A recent publication by Giuliani et al.,[20] is consistent with this observation. They measured the esophageal pressure-time product during synchronized intermittent mandatory ventilation and compared flow triggering versus pressure triggering and with constant flow versus constant pressure ventilation. As in other studies, they confirmed that flow triggering was associated with less effort than pressure triggering. In addition, they noted that this difference was greatest when flow triggering was associated with constant pressure ventilation.

Constant pressure ventilation is not new. It is identical to what was available in the Bennett "pressure" cycled ventilators (PR I and PR II) (Figure 1).

Other putative benefits of this mode, e.g., better distribution of ventilation remain to be documented and are of dubious value.

To recapitulate and summarize ventilator modes:

Controlled Ventilation: All ventilation is supplied by the mechanical ventilator. The patient makes no respiratory efforts. This mode is used only in paralyzed patients.

Assist-Control: The ventilator is set for a minimum number of breaths per minute, usually of a preset volume. Additional breaths may be initiated by the subject with a resultant preset volume delivered. This is probably the most commonly utilized mode. (This should be designated Volume Assisted, Assist-Control).

IMV: A preset number of machine breaths are delivered of a preset volume. Patient initiated breaths are unsupported. Beware of high resistance circuitry, which may be distressing to the patient.

Pressure Support Ventilation: In the strict definition, all breaths are initiated by the patient and the effort is supported with a preset supraatmospheric pressure. Putatively since the patient determines the pattern of airflow it is said to be "patient friendly." The preset pressure should be set to ensure patient comfort, which usually translates into a VT such that f is <25/minute.

IMV with Pressure Support: As above, all patient efforts are pressure supported but in addition there is a minimum backup machine rate and preset volume.

Pressure Controlled or Pressure-Preset Ventilation: All breaths, whether machine or patient initiated are delivered at a preset pressure in a square wave pattern. Since the peak pressure is present at the onset of inspiration, initial flows are high and tachypneic patients appear to be more comfortable than with other pressure waveforms. Other putative benefits remain to be proved. The P-$\dot{V}$ characteristics are identical to those seen with the Bennett PR II (Figure 1).

"Reverse Ratio" Ventilation: This should more appropriately be referred to as variable ratio, i.e., I:E, ventilation.[21] The emphasis is on

a prolonged inspiratory time at the expense of a shortened expiratory time. This may result in some increase in PaO_2 for a given FiO_2, which may be a consequence of an increase in mean alveolar pressure. Beware of barotrauma and cardiovascular compromise that may result from excessive PEEP.

CPAP: CPAP is not a mode for ventilating the lung. Rather it may be used as a weaning mode or as a substitute for a T tube trial prior to discontinuation of mechanical ventilation. Continuous flow CPAP requires less effort than non-continuous flow circuitry. In patients with intrinsic PEEP it may decrease the effort to initiate flow.[15]

To understand its appeal, let us again review the concept of intrinsic or auto-PEEP and its consequences. In patients with airways disease alveolar pressure at end-expiration may not return to atmospheric pressure as in the normal subject, i.e., alveolar pressure is supra-atmospheric or "positive" at end-expiration and this is referred to as auto-PEEP. Airflow cannot commence until alveolar pressure drops below atmospheric pressure. The addition of a positive pressure at the mouth is an effort to begin airflow from a mechanical source at a supra-atmospheric level, which approximates alveolar pressure and thus decreases inspiratory effort. Smith and Marini,[13] in fact, have shown experimentally that this may occur (Figure 6).

There are some reports that full face mask CPAP may in fact ease the effort of breathing in subjects who are acutely asthmatic, anecdotally reported to have averted intubation and ventilation.

There is, however, a much more practical and less theoretical reason for using this mode as a weaning mode. In some ventilators, e.g., Bennett 7200, the CPAP mode uses a continuous flow, which minimizes patient effort to initiate airflow and thus serves as a low resistance "blow by" comparable to a T price trial but without necessity for a change of equipment (see Weaning). This then reduces equipment costs and technician time.

Recently, a Canadian group has presented results from an initial clinical trial of what is referred to as "Proportional Assist Ventilation."[22,23] A rolling-seal piston is coupled to a motor that generates pressure in proportion to inspired flow and inspired volume so that proportionality between airway pressure and patient generated pressure was approximately 1:1. Proportional assist ventilation was tested in four normal subjects during heavy exercise and in five "stable ventilator dependent" patients recovering from "assorted medical disorders." The device responded to changes in patient effort with little delay and no impediment to gas movement from machine to patient, i.e., no valves to open. It was well tolerated and resulted in significant increase in patient's VT and decrease in f. This would appear to be a "patient friendly" system and has been compared to "variable ratio power steering." However, the first prototype was not "user friendly." Further, none of the patients had significant increases in airways resistance. This may prove to be an exciting addition to the ventilator management of patients with severe acute respiratory distress syndrome (ARDS). Its role in severe asthma with airflow limitation may be more problematic.

Ventilator Strategies

It is well to remember that mechanical ventilation is a support modality rather than a true therapeutic or curative modality. We support the patient with Guillain-Barre syndrome. In the asthmatic patient we do little more than protect the airway, and in the patient with ARDS we support oxygenation and try to protect other organ systems. It is humbling to recognize that the majority of patients who require mechanical ventilation for more than 7 days will not leave the hospital (exception are patients with neuromuscular disease).[24]

Imbued with this humility let me suggest that the most important dictum in the management of our ventilator patient is that we keep them comfortable. Remember that a patient breathing out of phase with a ventilator cannot be comfortable. Appreciate that such asynchrony may result in cardiovascular compromise and barotrauma. This leads to a corollary: "Keep the patient in phase with the ventilator." It is possible in the vast majority of patients to accomplish these goals without paralysis and/or deep narcosis. Many years ago, I was asked about the use of valium in ventilator management. I replied that valium should be spelled V-o-l-u-m-e. Patients with lung disease and respiratory failure all tend to breathe rapidly. In patients with diffuse lung disease, such as ARDS, fibrosis, or pulmonary edema, this behavior is thought to be due to exaggerated activity of lung stretch receptors. Hering and Breuer[25] in 1868, showed in the dog, cat, and rabbit, that expansion of the lung reflexly inhibited inspiration and promoted expiration. This effect depended upon the integrity of the vagus nerve. Curiously, this reflex in man has been demonstrated only under anesthesia. Further, Guz et al.[26] demonstrated in normal subjects under halothane anesthesia that inflation volumes of 1000 mL or more resulted in an inhibition of breathing. We believe that we have used this little appreciated observation to control the respiratory efforts of patients on mechanical ventilation and thus, "keep them in phase." We are now in a period where large lung volume breathing is being challenged.[27] We shall examine these fears relative to specific disease entities. Of additional interest is the response to lung deflation. Hering and Breuer[25] showed in the rabbit that reduction of lung volume arrests any expiratory activity and promptly elicits an inspiration. Subsequent studies by Troelstra and Widdicombe[25] confirm the fact that deflation of the lungs leads to an increase in frequency and force of the inspiratory effort. These observations may suggest a further rationale for the use of PEEP and may, in part, explain the beneficial effects of PEEP on lung water (see Chapter 1, Physiology, Applied) but as yet, have not been subjected to clinical scrutiny.

Neuromuscular Diseases

These patients are often cared for in specialty centers where efforts are often made to manage them without endotracheal intubation and non-invasive ventilator techniques. While this is a strategy for the long-term management of these patients, the acute episode, e.g., following spinal cord transection, is often associated with endotracheal secretions and/or pneumonia and usually requires intubation for airways management. In our institution, quadriplegics are managed by physical medicine and the preference is for large VT breathing, i.e., >15 mg/kg VT and rates between 8–12/minute. Ventilation of these patients is not a problem—weaning can be.

Cardiovascular Surgery and Pulmonary Edema

In our institution the majority of patients on ventilators are "postop hearts" and/or other "cardiacs," with systolic or diastolic dysfunction.

The vast majority of the post cardiovascular surgery patients are managed by protocol and extubated within 12 hours (see Weaning). However, a small number have persistent left ventricular dysfunction and require prolonged mechanical ventilation. As has been noted earlier in this textbook, a positive intrathoracic pressure may decrease left ventricular afterload[28] and be associated with an increase in cardiac output.[29,30] This concept has only recently been published and discussed in the clinical literature though it has been described for over 20 years in more basic science oriented publications.[31] Unfortunately it has been even slower to be incorporated into ventilator management of the cardiac patient with the failing heart. The publication of Lemaire et al.[32] and Permutt[33] is most instructive in this regard (Figure 7). The reports from Mathru et al.[29] and also Grace and Greenbaum[30] support the notion that a positive intrathoracic pressure may be beneficial in the patient with left ventricular dysfunction with or without pulmonary edema. These observations have led us to adopt a strategy of "controlled ventilation" for these patients and, in fact, we use PEEP liberally. However, unlike the patient with ARDS, where oxygenation is a major problem and often dictates PEEP strategies, the goal in these subjects is to optimize cardiac performance, i.e., decrease filling pressures and increase cardiac output.

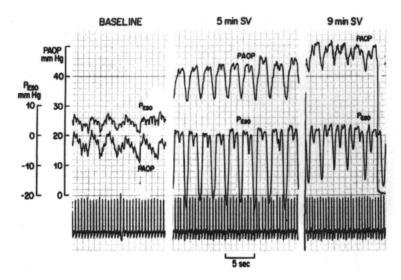

Figure 7. Mechanical ventilation. Upon removal from mechanical ventilation esophageal pressure becomes subatmospheric (negative) and PA wedge pressure promptly rises. (Reprinted with permission from Ref. 32.)

Maintain a positive intrathoracic pressure until volume status and cardiac performance is judged to be optimal, then and only then do we attempt to withdraw the ventilator (see Weaning).

Asthma

The best strategy for the asthmatic patient, if at all possible, is to avoid intubation and ventilation. Do not intubate simply because of hypercarbia. Remember that hypercarbia per se does not kill and that intubation and ventilation does not guarantee eucarbia.[34] Recall also, that most asthmatics with hypercarbia will be eucarbic within 8 hours and over 90% within 24 hours.[35] The principal dictum in the management of the patient in status asthmaticus is "deflate the lung." Hyperinflation is associated with auto-PEEP, which in turn increases the work of breathing, leads to an increased respiratory rate, a decreased expiratory time, and further hyperinflation and auto-PEEP, and ultimately cardiovascular compromise.[36] In our institution, we willingly administer a trial of morphine before intubation and ventilation. The goal is to slow the rate, increase expiratory time, and decrease auto-PEEP. Curiously, this therapeutic maneuver is usually not associated with an increase in Pa_{CO_2}. Remember that rapid f is associated with a disproportionate distribution of ventilation to lung zones with high

VA/Qc ratios, i.e., wasted ventilation (Figures 8 and 9).[37] In other institutions, attempts have been made to match the patients auto-PEEP with CPAP by full face mask. Beneficial results have been reported. In all probability application of CPAP required morphine or other sedation.

The indication for intubation then should be a sense of impending doom. The airway must be protected. Remember that the goal is not to achieve eucarbia. Eucarbia will occur as the asthma improves, usually within 24 hours. There are three goals: (1) maintain oxygenation (rarely a problem); (2) avoid barotrauma; and (3) deflate the lung.

The reader is referred to the excellent series of articles from Tuxen's group.[36,38,39] The basic principles to be taken away from these papers are:

High pressures per se do not cause barotrauma. Barotrauma is related to the degree of air trapping.[36]

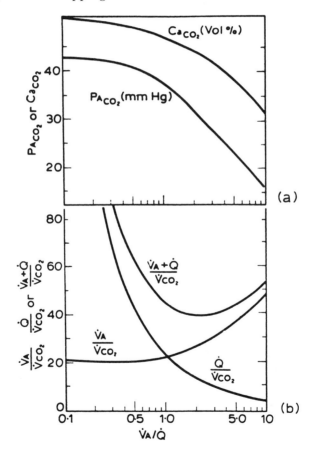

Figure 8. Effect of VA/Q on CO_2 transport. Top half—effect on alveolar capillary tensions and capillary CO_2 content. Bottom half—flow requirements. (Reprinted with permission from Ref. 37.)

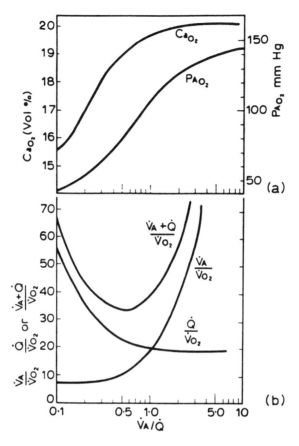

Figure 9. Effect of VA/Q on O_2 transport. Both halves pertain to normal resting conditions and have VA/Q on a log scale for abscissa. In the top half the effects on Pao_2 and on the capillary blood oxygen saturation are shown. In the bottom half the ventilatory requirement, perfusion requirement, and total flow requirement for O_2 uptake are shown. In Figures 8 and 9, focus on the curves VA/VCO_2 and VA/VO_2. These are expressions of efficiency of gas exchange. An increase in Va without an increase in blood flow results in high VA/QC ratios. Note the optimum ratio for O_2 and CO_2 exchange lies between 0.5 and 1.0. Higher ratios represent "wasted ventilation" or costly ventilation. (Reprinted with permission from Ref. 37.)

To deflate the lung and reduce air trapping allow a long expiratory time. The corollaries of this are: Choose a slow respiratory rate and a very short inspiratory time, i.e., high inspiratory flow rates that in turn require very high peak pressures. Recall that the major source of airways resistance in acute decompensated asthma, unlike COPD, probably exists in proximal airways[40] in addition to peripheral airways, and that acute asthma tends to be a symmetrical disease. Asymmetric hyperinflation

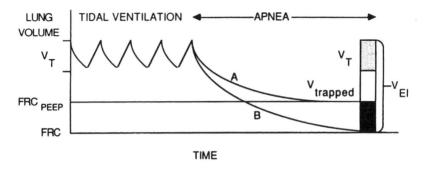

Figure 10. Mechanical ventilation.(Reprinted with permission from Ref. 38.)

and barotrauma associated with high pressure, per se, was not noted by Williams.36

The initial VT will of necessity be small because of ventilator limits, e.g., 5–8 mL/kg.

As the asthma improves and trapped gas decreases, increase minute volume till eucarbia is achieved. This requires frequent observations and increase in VT. When eucarbia is achieved without paralysis, the patient is usually ready for extubation (see Weaning).

To follow this protocol may require deep sedation and even paralyzing agents. Tuxen et al.[39] routinely use paralyzing agents and then follow the trapped air after a 40-second apneic phase (Figure 10). We rarely paralyze patients and prefer to substitute a surrogate for trapped gas, i.e., auto-PEEP as an index of air trapping. Remember that paradoxical pulse may also be a good clinical indicator of auto-PEEP. This can often be appreciated by two fingers on the femoral artery.

Remember then: (1) avoid barotrauma; and (2) deflate the lung.

If paralysis is required it can usually be discontinued within 24 hours. The vast majority of these patients should be extubated within 24 to 48 hours (see Weaning).

COPD

Depending upon how much these patients tend to be asthmatic or primarily emphysema, will determine the difficulty or ease with which they may be managed. The principles are the same as for the asthmatics. Expiratory time must be long and respiratory rate ca 8–12/minute so as to prevent development of intrinsic PEEP.

Tracheobronchial secretions are often what necessitates intubation and ventilation rather than severe bronchospasm unless, of course, the subject is an asthmatic.

Except in those patients who are terminal, the outcome tends to be favorable.[41] If possible, patients who are terminal should not be subjected to the trauma of intubation and ventilation. However, this is a judgment that is best made by a caring primary care physician and a loving family. An intensivist who sees such a patient for the first time is at a distinct disadvantage and demonstrates why the primary physician must not be excluded from the loop. Remember that a physician is not obligated to participate in therapy that is futile. Also recall that patients can live with Pa_{CO_2}'s of 60–80 torr and often higher if oxygenation is maintained. The kidney is capable of generating a serum HCO_3 of about 45 meq so that for a Pa_{CO_2} of 80 and HCO_3 of 48 the pH will be 7.40. Also, the Bohr equation tends to stabilize the Pa_{CO_2} so that CO_2 generated each minute is eliminated with less alveolar ventilation at a higher set point. Bohr equation:

$$\dot{V}_{CO_2} = \dot{V}_A \bullet FA_{CO_2}. \qquad FA_{CO_2} = Pa_{CO_2}/P_B$$
$$or\,\dot{V}_{CO_2} = \dot{V}_A \bullet Pa_{CO_2}/P_B \tag{1}$$

Thus, a patient with a Pa_{CO_2} of 70 is in equilibrium with her CO_2 production with half the alveolar ventilation of a subject with a Pa_{CO_2} of 35.

Should a patient with terminal emphysema be intubated, extubation can be a nightmare (see Weaning). Remember that before engaging in aggressive therapeutic intervention primum dictum non nocere. An alternative strategy is suggested in the reports of Brochard et al.[42,43]

Previously, Brochard and colleagues[42] had proposed that patients with COPD and respiratory failure might be ventilated with non-invasive pressure support ventilation delivered through a face mask. Recently, they demonstrated in a prospective randomized study that non-invasive ventilation of patients with acute exacerbations of COPD could reduce the need for endotracheal intubation, length of hospital stay, and in-hospital mortality rate.[43] This is reminiscent of strategies utilized in the mid and late 1950s and, in an era of cost containment and ethical concerns about prolongation of dying, should receive thoughtful consideration. Results with nasal mask ventilation have been less encouraging and in our experience, relatively ineffective and troublesome to patients and personnel.

ARDS

There is probably no greater challenge in the practice of critical care medicine than the ventilator management of patients with acute lung injury or the ARDS. These terms are generally considered to be synonymous except for a slight difference in oxygenation parameters. The syndrome is characterized by a chest x ray, which demonstrates diffuse bilateral lung infiltrates, a pulmonary artery occlusion pressure <19 mmHg or no clinical evidence of left atrial hypertension and a significant degree of arterial hypoxemia, i.e., PaO_2/FiO_2 ratio of <200 regardless of the amount of PEEP.[44]

The pathology in the first 5 days is associated with a protein rich pulmonary edema and atelectasis and an infiltration of acute inflammatory cells. As the process progresses inflammations and fibrosis dominates the patho-anatomy.[45,46]

In its purest form, the syndrome is seen with sepsis and the lung injury is secondary to a multitude of factors, which include neutrophils, mononuclear cells, endotoxin, and other sepsis related mediators and finally to the abnormal response of pulmonary endothelial and epithelial cells. The exact role of surfactant secretion is unclear.

In addition to sepsis, this syndrome may also result from fat emboli or from direct endobronchial insults, such as aspiration of gastric contents. Diffuse, five-lobe pneumonia may also be seen with influenza A infection and infrequently with other infectious etiologies.

Typically, the patient manifests tachypnea and tachycardia and severe arterial hypoxemia relatively resistant to oxygen breathing. Since the syndrome was popularized by Ashbaugh et al.[1] about 30 years ago, it has become customary to intubate and ventilate these subjects. PEEP was popularized by Ashbaugh et al.[1] to decrease intrapulmonary shunting and improve oxygenation and thus, decrease the requirements for supplemental oxygen.

Mortality in this syndrome has characteristically been in excess of 50% and may approach 100% in patients with multiple organ failure (MOF).[47,48] Three organ failure for more than 7 days is associated with 98% mortality.[47] In fact, the vast majority of deaths are attributable to MOF and the underlying disease process. Infrequently, death is due to progressive respiratory failure.[48] Clearly, it is difficult to reach a consensus as to the optimum strategy for ventilator support in ARDS. However, there is growing concern that ARDS is to a significant degree, iatrogenic[27] and it has even been suggested that MOF may be related to mediators released from the injured lung,[49] which is further traumatized by mechanical ventilation and/or O_2.

In 1965, Castleman used the term respirator lung in the discussion of a clinico-pathologic conference in the New England Journal of Medicine.[50] Cosentino[51] suggested that the lung pathology might be due to deleterious effects of oxygen and referred to Morgan et al.[52] Shortly thereafter, Nash et al.[53] from the Massachusetts General Hospital, published their sentinel paper that incriminated a high FiO_2 as the cause of lung damage. However, early on, there was evidence that ventilation per se could interfere with surfactant production and lead to lung instability.[54] Subsequent clinical literature has failed to confirm the toxic effects of O_2 in the management of ARDS.[55,56] Experimental data, however, suggests it is prudent to limit FiO_2.[57] Consensus conference suggests FiO <0.6.[19] PEEP has been advocated early on to improve oxygenation and reduce FiO_2 and has been recognized that it may be associated with barotrauma, i.e., pneumothorax and pneumomediastinum. Further, ARDS, as currently managed, i.e., VT of 10–15 mL/kg, "normalize" pH and Pco_2 without attempt to limit airway pressures, may put the injured lung at risk for further damage.[19] It is known that the pulmonary pathology of ARDS is not homogeneously distributed and only a fraction of the lung is ventilated with each breath. The apparent low compliance may in fact be lung volume related rather than a true "stiff lung."[58] Further, there is a vertical gradient of lung inflation, i.e., dependent zones manifest a decrease in inflation and an increase in CT density.[59] Thus, during conventional ventilatory management of ARDS, the bulk of ventilation may be directed to less involved units with potentially harmful over distension. However, before we adopt a strategy of small VT breathing, let us not forget the atelectatic areas in the more dependent lung zones. A recent paper by Muscedere et al.[60] suggests that lung units ventilated with a PEEP level below the critical opening pressure demonstrated significant lung injury. Also, some studies that have compared high frequency oscillatory (HFO) ventilation with conventional ventilation have reported a lower incidence of barotrauma.[61] These studies have utilized a strategy of aggressive volume recruitment and mean airway pressures have been higher than with conventional ventilation.[62,63] Benefits have been attributed to avoidance of lower lung volumes and smaller pressure-volume changes.[61,64] However, the HIFI multicenter, randomized trial failed to demonstrate any benefit of HFO ventilation over conventional ventilation in preterm infants.[65] It would appear that the lung must be recruited but that it is prudent to avoid over distension. Dreyfuss and Saumon[66] have referred to this dilemma as being between the Charybdis and the Scylla, those two immortal and irresistible monsters of Greek mythology who beset the Straits of Messina between Calabria, Italy, and Sicily.

"Open the lung and keep it open."[67] What is optimal PEEP? The work of Suter et al.[68] is worth revisiting. Their data suggest that in normovolemic patient, total static compliance is a simple and useful means of finding the degree of lung distension that provides the best gas exchange with the least risk of alveolar over distension and lung rupture. In their study, arterial oxygen transport and whole body $avDo_2$ were also found to be optimal at that level of PEEP.

Another strategy designed to recruit alveolar units, but limit plateau pressure, has been referred to as inverse ratio ventilation.[21] This should more appropriately be termed variable ratio I:E ventilation. The object is to recruit alveolar units by increasing inspiratory time but to avoid an increase in PEEP.[69] Small increases in PaO_2 have been reported but no study has demonstrated improved outcome.[70] This intervention, in our experience, has proved to be labor intensive and was abandoned several years ago. The publication of Lessard et al.[70] demonstrated no benefit of inverse ratio ventilation versus conventional ventilation with PEEP and, in fact, may result in significant decrease in cardiac output and O_2 delivery.[71,72]

There are reports from New Zealand by Hickling et al.[73] that suggests improved survival in ARDS managed with low volume, pressure-limited ventilation with permissive hypercapnia and hypoxemia. PaO_2 was often in the 50s. However, these studies were not controlled and must be repeated. Unexplained is that even the presence of MOF was associated with improved outcome. They suggested that MOF may be related to lung injury and release of injurious mediators and that the remarkably good outcomes in their series was associated with, and due to, less lung trauma.

If we are responsible for iatrogenic lung injury in ARDS, we must ask is it volutrauma or barotrauma? The work of Dreyfuss et al.[74,75] suggests the culprit is high volume and not pressure per se and in fact, that PEEP has a protective effect on permeability lung edema. Curiously the animals ventilated with negative inspiratory pressure had the greatest degrees of edema, a lesson to be remembered when a significant number of patients' breaths on a ventilator may be spontaneous as in the IMV mode or partially supported as in IMV with pressure support, wherein Ppl may be significantly negative.

The awareness that we may be doing harm in ARDS has led some to reconsider HFO and extracorporeal CO_2 removal.[76] However, their beneficial effects in ARDS remain unproven. Minimally invasive adjuncts such as intracorporeal CO_2 removal by an IV oxygenator or by insufflation of gas into the trachea to reduce dead space ventilation remain to be tested.[77]

The role of surfactant in ARDS is unclear but certainly very expensive. Intratracheal perfluorocarbon[78] also reduces alveolar surface tension and may prove to be an attractive alternative to surfactant therapy.

Might the time be appropriate to reconsider whether patients with ARDS should be mechanically ventilated? Graziano Carlon, in the 1980s, believed that the mainstay of therapy for ARDS was PEEP and this led him to his extensive research on HFO ventilation that culminated in an "International Symposium on HFV" sponsored by Memorial Sloan-Kettering Cancer Center, New York, 1983. Note that variable ratio I:E ventilation comparable to HFO increases mean alveolar pressure but limits peak and plateau pressures. The most recent "wrinkle" on this strategy proposed by Downs and collaborator[79] is referred to as "airway pressure release ventilation" (APRV). This technique basically consists of CPAP created by a high gas flow to the breathing circuit to maintain a nearly constant level of CPAP during spontaneous respiration. The increase in functional residual capacity is thought to be the basis for the observed benefits. Intermittently CPAP is interrupted to promote CO_2 elimination. Hickling et al's.[73] observations would suggest this need not occur frequently. A prospective multicenter trial was conducted and it was concluded that APRV is a feasible alternative to conventional ventilation in acute lung injury of mild to moderate severity.[80]

The studies of Hickling et al.[73] remind us that patients with ARDS infrequently die as a result of respiratory failure unless we choose to discontinue mechanical ventilation. The recognition that the problem in sepsis and ARDS is at a tissue level reemphasizes the need to examine oxygen utilization. Patients with sepsis and ARDS often have an increased cardiac output, a low peripheral vascular resistance and a well preserved mixed venous oxygen saturation. Raising the arterial Po_2 as with the addition of PEEP has not increased survival in ARDS.[81] An alternate strategy to increase peripheral oxygen utilization was suggested by the early report of Danek et al.[82] who reported that oxygen utilization was dependent on oxygen delivery in ARDS. In normal individuals O_2 utilization is dependent upon delivery only below a certain critical level (Figure 11).

Thus it was reasoned that increasing delivery to supranormal levels (i.e., supranormal levels, i.e., Do_2 >600 mL/minute, cardiac index >4.5 L/minute per m_2 body-surface area and O_2 consumption >170 mL/minute per square meter body-surface area) might have a favorable influence on survival. In their study O_2 consumption was not measured independently because of the many problems associated with this measurement in a critically ill patient in the ICU. Rather O_2 consumption was calculated from measurements of cardiac output and arteriovenous oxygen difference (Fick equation). Thus, the measurement of oxygen consumption was in fact directly related to the variable with which it was being compared, i.e., cardiac output. Studies by Shoemaker et al.[83,84] in high risk surgical patients and in patients with severe trauma also suggest that increased O_2 delivery to supranormal level is associated with a more favorable outcome. In most of their subjects their therapeutic goals were achieved with fluid resuscitation alone and without need for pressors and/or isotropic agents. Utilizing a slightly different study design, two reports from London show no benefit from increasing Do_2 to supranormal levels with dobutamine.[85,86] Noteworthy is that subjects who achieved hemodynamic goals with fluid administration alone were not randomly assigned to the treatment or control group and all survived to leave the hospital.

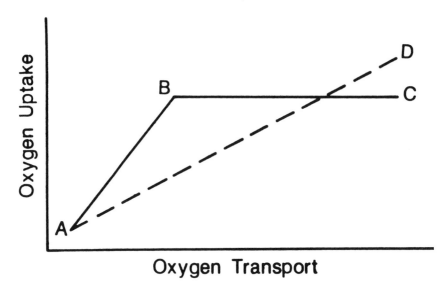

Figure 11. Mechanical ventilation. O_2 uptake versus O_2 transport. Note that the broken line AD believed by some to represent the situation in sepsis and/or ARDS has not been documented by others. See text. From : Dantzker, Cardio-Pulmonary Critical Care (2nd ed.), W. B. Saunders, p. 659, Fig. 20–1, 1991. (Reprinted with permission from W. B. Saunders Co.)

Where are we at present? In the absence of good data, there is a consensus statement that plateau pressure should be maintained below 35 cm H_2O. PEEP levels should probably be used in the range of 10–15 cm H_2O and FiO_2 should not exceed 0.6. Many of these patients have an increased cardiac output and the limiting factor in tissue oxygenation may be a peripheral shunt rather than arterial hypoxemia.

Though the waters are murky, patient comfort must be ensured. Strategies include sedation, higher ventilator rates to attempt to match the patient and probably a VT of 5–10 mL/kg. A plateau pressure of <35 cm H_2O is to be preferred but may not be achievable and should not become the standard of care until more data are available. FiO_2 should not exceed 0.6. O_2 transport should take precedence over Sao_2. However, supranormal oxygen delivery in ARDS has not been associated with increased survival. Prolonged paralysis should be avoided. The reports from Miller's group at the University of California/San Francisco of prolonged paralysis after vecuronium is sobering.[87] A patient who is likely to die should be permitted a chance to relate to friends and relatives while receiving our too often futile ministrations.

Weaning

To accustom a child or young animal to food other than its mother's milk; to free from a habit or attitude.[88]

When, if ever, is weaning required, i.e., the gradual removal of ventilatory support? At one end of the spectrum is the subject who is intubated, paralyzed, and ventilated during general anesthesia for an operative procedure. When the patient is awake and has return of muscle function, ventilation can be safely terminated and the endotracheal tube removed. A comparable situation probably exists in the case of a patient with hypertensive cardiovascular disease who develops a sudden episode of pulmonary edema (flash pulmonary edema). After adequate diuresis and control of hypertension, extubation can usually be accomplished without an intermediate period of gradual decrease in ventilatory support. More problematic are patients who require mechanical ventilator support because of intrinsic lung disease, i.e., airways disease or ARDS, or because of potentially reversible neuromuscular disease. Must these patients be weaned and if so, which ones, or do we simply provide support until they are capable of independent breathing? That is, does the weaning process of itself contribute to improvement in respiratory status?

The statement of the ATS is worth reading and reflecting upon and several excerpts are stated here[89]: "Only about 5% of patients who are mechanically ventilated cannot be successfully removed from machine support on the first and second attempt." "Although only a small minority of patients present true problems in weaning from mechanical ventilation, these same patients consume a disproportionate share of acute care resources."[89]

A historical review may help us to better understand why "weaning" in many institutions has become a routine part of ventilator care even in the absence of good supporting data.

Early efforts in respiratory care often used so-called pressure cycled ventilators. The prescription often amounted to a form of pressure support ventilation. The patient's own efforts usually determined the respiratory rate. A machine set rate was simply a "back up" rate. It was a natural that the entire therapeutic strategy should be one of declining support as the patient's respiratory status improved. At some point, usually when lung mechanics, i.e., vital capacity and/or maximum inspiratory force and oxygenation were considered, adequate T tube trials were instituted and clinical observations were supplemented with arterial blood gas analysis.

Such trials were often lengthy although pioneers in the field like Dr. Tom Petty often cautioned against long trials. Often the patients were placed back on mechanical ventilation at night and then T tube trials resumed during daytime hours. Clearly the period on the T tube was regarded as a therapeutic exercise. "The respiratory muscles were being reconditioned," a curious notion since early theories of respiratory failure implicated respiratory muscle fatigue as the indication for intubation and ventilation. It would seem to follow that the muscles should be rested and not exercised.

"Although a significant body of data indicates that training maneuvers improve performance in stable patients and normal subjects, very little data are available to confirm that similar principles apply to the critically ill patient."[89]

In the late 1960s, Kirby et al.[5] introduced IMV as a means of utilizing high levels of PEEP for the treatment of ARDS. Emphasized in this strategy were the spontaneous breaths rather than the mandatory mechanical breaths. During patient powered inspiration, venous return was promoted so as to counter the effects of PEEP on venous return and cardiac output. IMV was quickly accepted by many as a "weaning mode" intended to replace the "swim or sink" approach of the T tube trials. Curiously though, no study ever demonstrated superiority of IMV versus T tube trials as a weaning mode—the proponents of IMV were not to be deterred. In fact, because of the ventilator circuitry in many IMV modes, the work of breathing for the patients was significantly increased compared with the T tube.[6] Did this increased work enhance respiratory muscle function or in fact, perpetrate respiratory muscle fatigue? Most of the data would favor the latter.

This, then, led to the development of IMV with pressure support.[11] During the subject initiated breath, mechanical support was applied. It would appear we had come full circle. As noted earlier in this section, this mode of ventilation in its pressure flow characteristics was essentially identical to the performance of the Bennett PR II pressure flow cycled ventilator. The pressures used in the original investigation of this mode, IMV plus pressure support, approximated those used with the machine initiated breaths. The putative benefit of this mode was that patients could tailor the flow pattern and thus should be more comfortable. In fact, in the first report, patients were more comfortable, a not unexpected finding since one essentially compared unassisted ventilation with assisted ventilation.

Nevertheless, the question remained: did IMV with pressure support facilitate discontinuation of mechanical ventilation in patients with respiratory failure and if so, in which subsets of patients, i.e., airways disease, ARDS, or left ventricular failure?

Only one paper to date suggests a superiority of IMV with pressure support over assist-control ventilation with intermittent T tube trials.[90] However, a more recent publication from the Spanish Lung Failure Collaborative Group[91] showed that assist-control ventilation with once daily brief (up to 2 hours) T tube trials was superior to IMV and to IMV with pressure support as a means to discontinue ventilator support in a selected group of patients who were judged to be difficult to extubate. This group comprised 132 patients who demonstrated poor tolerance during the initial trial of spontaneous breathing. This group made up 24% of the total group who required mechanical ventilation, i.e., 76% were extubated without "weaning."

There are several lessons to be learned from these reports. First, at least three-quarters of all ventilated subjects are ready to be extubated after a brief trial of spontaneous ventilation without a prolonged period of gradually diminishing ventilator support. Second, it is problematic whether any subjects are truly weaned. The length of time from the initiation of "weaning" to successful extubation in the Spanish group was 1–6 days, median 3 days, in those given a once daily trial of spontaneous breathing (up to 2 hours). The total time spent in the weaning mode was 2–12 hours, a length of time unlikely to favorably influence lung and respiratory muscle mechanics. On the other hand, in the Brochard et al.[90] series, T tube trials of 2 hours each were sometimes used three times daily. Further, before being extubated, patients had to tolerate an IMV rate of 4/minute for at least 24 hours before being extubated, a considerable ventilatory challenge. Might this strategy have caused continued muscle fatigue or have contributed to lung water?[32]

Until now, in this chapter, I have discussed "weaning modes and strategies." The reader may ask, "But when does weaning begin?" or in my opinion more appropriately, "When can mechanical ventilation be terminated?" Over the years, various criteria have been examined, some very simple and others much more complex. These have included vital capacity, VT, f, maximum inspiratory force, minute ventilation versus maximum voluntary ventilation, occlusion mouth pressures with and without hypercarbic challenge and adequacy of arterial blood gas analysis. All, with the exception of f and VT have been found lacking in sensitively and specificity. Yang and Tobin[92] showed that the ratio of f/VT is the best at predicting failure or success for discontinuation of mechanical ventilation, so that a ratio of >100 predicts failure and if <100, success (Figure 12).[90]

Yang and Tobin[92] demonstrated that this simple ratio was superior to a more complex CROP index. The CROP included measures of compliance, rate, oxygenation, and pressure. Again, in this study, those patients with a favorable "weaning index" were extubated after a brief T tube trial without further weaning techniques (personal communication). It would seem then, that these criteria would more appropriately be designated as criteria for discontinuation of mechanical ventilation rather than weaning criteria.

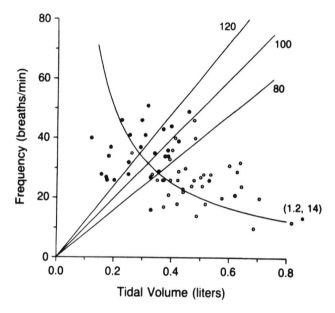

Figure 12. Weaning from mechanical ventilation. ○ = weaned successfully; • = failed to wean. (Reprinted with permission from Ref. 92.)

Further, Tobin et al.[93] have shown that those subjects who are not ready for extubation will demonstrate a high f low VT pattern of breathing almost immediately upon cessation of mechanical support thus lending credibility to the short trial without support. The exception to this based upon our experience is the patient with poor left ventricular function. In these subjects, the ventilator may be serving as a cardiac assist.[31,32] In such patients, the pulmonary capillary wedge pressure will rise in minutes but respiratory decompensation may be delayed, though admittedly in Lemaire's[32] subjects respiratory distress was noted early in the erratic behavior of the esophageal pressure tracings. In the absence of a PA line, a 20% increase in pulse rate or a drop in blood pressure could similarly reflect poor left ventricular function. We proceed more cautiously with these subjects, e.g., T tube trials up to 2 hours and frequent observations. "A large percentage of patients who repeatedly fail to wean from mechanical ventilation have overt or occult heart failure."[89]

A few comments are appropriate about the ventilator or T tube circuitry during observation of the patient believed to be ready for extubation. While the T tube circuitry is most simple, it requires a change of equipment and technician time. Therefore, in many units, patients are asked to breathe through the ventilator without mechanical assistance. It behooves the physician to be familiar with the circuitry and the resistances therein. CPAP is often a part of the prescription. Recognize that CPAP for all practical purposes does not give a respiratory assist in the usual manner of thinking about respiratory assistance, i.e., a supra-atmospheric pressure above the end-expiratory pressure applied to the airway during inspiration. In patients with persistently positive airways pressure at end-expiration, i.e., intrinsic PEEP, the addition of an equal or lesser amount of PEEP in the form of CPAP may lessen the effort required to initiate a breath.[15] Once initiated, however, the resistance that the patient must overcome to maintain flow can be significant. In other words, not all CPAP modes are created equally.[16] Some ventilators in the CPAP mode have a continuous flow of air, e.g., Bennett 7200, which minimizes resistance to breathing. It has been shown that resistance is less in continual flow CPAP circuits.[16]

Sassoon[94] compared three "weaning modes", T tube, IMV, and CPAP5 with continuous flow (Bennett 7200) and measured the time-pressure product. She found it to be least with the CPAP5-cm H_2O, continuous flow. However, all patients were successfully extubated, which suggested the differences were clinically insignificant.[94]

Which mode you choose seems to make little difference for a short period of observation, i.e., <2 hours, caveat. If a patient you believe can be extubated fails a period of observation, check the circuitry. A T tube with high flow is still the least complex and the time tested standard.

In summary, the majority of patients who require mechanical ventilation can be extubated after brief "blow by" trials if the observed f/VT ratio is <100. I recommend that these measurements be made daily. Asthmatic subjects should be ready for extubation within 24–48 hours. Patients with ARDS additionally must be able to maintain a reasonable level of oxygenation without PEEP and with an FiO_2 <0.60. What is considered a reasonable level of oxygenation will be a function of cardiac output. For a young person with a 10 L cardiac output a Pao_2 >55 torr may suffice. Subjects who repeatedly fail "blow by" trials or who deteriorate late, i.e., after 2 hours on "blow by" are often in congestive heart failure and may actually deteriorate as a result of weaning trials, which result in subatmospheric intrapleural pressures. Whether the actual process of gradually withdrawing ventilatory support, i.e., weaning, results in facilitation of withdrawal of mechanical support is controversial. The recent report of the Spanish Collaborative study would suggest that subjects with respiratory failure do best if fully supported until the disease process heals and at that point ventilation may be abruptly terminated without gradual withdrawal of support, i.e., fledging.

FLEDGE: To raise a young bird until it is able to fly.[95]

References

1. Ashbaugh DC, Bigelow DB, Petty TL. Acute respiratory distress in adults. Lancet 1967;2:319–323.
2. Banner MJ, Lampotang S, Boysen PC, et al. Flow resistance of expiratory positive-pressure valve systems. Chest 1986;90:212–217.
3. Marini JJ, Culver BH, Kirk W. Flow resistance of exhalation valves and positive end-expiratory pressure devices used in mechanical ventilation. Am Rev Respir Dis 1985;131:850–854.
4. Pinsky MR, Hrehochik D, Culpepper JA, et al. Flow resistance of expiratory positive pressure systems. Chest 1988;94:788–791.
5. Kirby RR, Downs JB, Civetta J, et al. High level PEEP in acute respiratory insufficiency. Chest 1975;67:156–163.
6. Gibney RT, Wilson RS, Pontoppidan H. Comparison of work of breathing on high gas flow and demand valve continuous positive airway pressure systems. Chest 1982;6:692–695.
7. Marini JJ, Rodriguez RM, Lamb V. Inspiratory workload of patient initiated mechanical ventilation. Am Rev Respir Dis 1986;134:902–909.
8. Hillman K, Friedlos J, Davey A. A comparison of intermittent mandatory ventilation systems. Crit Care Med 1986;14:499–502.
9. Marini JJ, Capps JS, Culver BH. The inspiratory work of breathing during assisted mechanical ventilation. Chest 1985;87:612–618.
10. Christopher KL, Neff TA, Bowman JL, et al. Demand and continuous flow intermittent mandatory ventilation systems. Chest 1985;87:625–630.
11. MacIntyre NR. Respiratory function during pressure support ventilation. Chest 1986;89:677–683.
12. Pepe PE, Marini JJ. Occult positive end-expiratory pressure in mechanically ventilated patients with airflow obstruction. The auto-PEEP effect. Am Rev Respir Dis 1982;126:166–170.
13. Smith TC, Marini JJ. Impact of PEEP on lung mechanics and work of breathing in severe airflow obstruction. J Appl Physiol 1988;65(4):1488–1499.
14. Tuxen DV. Detrimental effects of positive end-expiratory pressure during controlled mechanical ventilation of patients with severe airflow obstruction. Am Rev Respir Dis 1989;140:5–9.
15. Petrof BJ, Legare M, Goldberg P, et al. Continuous positive airway pressure reduced work of breathing and dyspnea during weaning from mechanical ventilation in severe chronic obstructive pulmonary disease. Am Rev Respir Dis 1990;141:281–289.
16. Samodelov LF, Falke KJ. Total inspiratory work with modern demand valve devices compared to continuous flow CPAC. Int Care Med 1988;14:632–639.
17. Marini JJ, Crooke PS, Truwit JD. Determinants and limits of pressure-preset ventilation: A mathematical model of pressure control. J Appl Physiol 1989;67:1081–1092.
18. Brochard L, Pluskwa F, Lemaire F. Improved efficacy of spontaneous breathing with inspiratory pressure support. Am Rev Respir Dis 1987;136:411–415.
19. Consensus Conference on Mechanical Ventilation, January 28–30, 1993. Int Care Med 1994;20:64–79.
20. Giuliani R, Mascia L, Recchia F, et al. Patient-ventilator interaction during synchronized IMV. Effects of flow triggering. Am J Respir Crit Care Med 1995;151:1–9.

21. Marcy TW, Marini JJ. Increase-ratio ventilation in ARDS; rationale and implementation. Chest 1991;100:494–504.
22. Younes M. Proportional assist ventilation: A new approach to ventilatory support. Am Rev Respir Dis 1992;145:114–120.
23. Younes M, Pudry A, Roberts D, et al. Proportional assist ventilation: Results of an initial clinical trial. Am Rev Respir Dis 1992;145:121–129.
24. Knaus WA. Prognosis with mechanical ventilation. The influence of disease, severity of disease, age and chronic health status on survival from an acute illness. Am Rev Respir Dis 1989;140:S8–S13.
25. Breathing. Hering-Breuer Centenary Symposium, Porter R (ed). Ciba Foundation, 1970.
26. Guz A, Noble MIM, Eisele JH, et al. Role of vagal inflation reflexes in man and other animals. Hering-Breuer Centenary Symposium, Porter R (ed). Ciba Foundation, 1970.
27. Marini JJ. Re-targeting ventilatory objectives in adult respiratory distress syndrome. New treatment prospects—persistent questions. Am Rev Respir Dis 1992;146:2–3.
28. Buda AJ, Pinsky MR, Ingels NB, et al. Effect of intrathoracic pressure on left ventricular performance. N Engl J Med 1979;301:453–459.
29. Mathru M, Rao TL, El-Etr AA, et al. Hemodynamic responses to changes in ventilatory patterns in patients with normal and poor left ventricular reserve. Crit Care Med 1982;10:423–426.
30. Grace MP, Greenbaum DM. Cardiac performance in response to PEEP in patients with cardiac dysfunction. Crit Care Med 1982;10:358–360.
31. Pinsky MR, Summer WR, Wise RA, et al. Augmentation of cardiac function by elevation of intrathoracic pressure. J Appl Physiol 1983;54:950–955.
32. Lemaire F, Teboul J-L, Cinotti L, et al. Acute left ventricular dysfunction during unsuccessful weaning from mechanical ventilation. Anesthesiology 1988;69:171–179.
33. Permutt S. Circulatory effects of weaning from mechanical ventilation: The importance of transdiaphragmatic pressure. Anesthesthesiology 1988;69:157–160.
34. Darioli R, Perret C. Mechanical controlled hypoventilation in status asthmaticus. Am Rev Respir Dis 1984;129:385–387.
35. Scoggin CH, Sahn SA, Petty TL. Status asthmaticus: A nine-year experience. JAMA 1977;238:1158–1162.
36. Williams TJ, Tuxen DV, Scheinkestel CO, et al. Risk factors for morbidity in mechanically ventilated patients with acute severe asthma. Am Rev Respir Dis 1992;146:607–615.
37. Farhi LE. Ventilation-perfusion relationship and its role in alveolar gas exchange. In: Caro CG (ed). Advances in Respiratory Physiology. Williams & Wilkins, 1966.
38. Tuxen DV, Lane S. Effects of ventilatory pattern on hyperinflation, airway pressures and circulation in mechanical ventilation of patients with severe air-flow obstruction. Am Rev Respir Dis 1987;136:872–879.
39. Tuxen DV, Williams TJ, Scheinkestel CD, et al. Use of measurement of pulmonary hyperinflation to control the level on mechanical ventilation in patients with acute severe asthma. Am Rev Respir Dis 1992;146:1136–1142.
40. Macklem PJ, Despas PJ, Leroux M. Site of airway obstruction in asthma. 1973;Chest 63(Suppl):28S.
41. Hudson LD. Survival data in patients with an acute and chronic lung disease requiring mechanical ventilation. Am Rev Respir Dis 1989;140:S19–S24.

42. Brochard L, Isabey D, Piquet J, et al. Reversal of acute exacerbations of chronic obstructive lung disease by inspiratory assistance with a face mask. N Engl J Med 1990;323:1523–1530.
43. Brochard L, Mancebo J, Wysocki M, et al. Non-invasive ventilation for acute exacerbations of chronic obstructive pulmonary disease. N Engl J Med 1995;333: 817–822.
44. The American-European Consensus Conference on ARDS (Definitions, Mechanisms, Relevant Outcomes, and Clinical Trial Coordination). Participants: Bernard GR, Artigas A, Brigham KL, et al. Am J Respir Crit Care Med 1994;149: 818–824.
45. Katzenstein ALA, Bloor CM, Liebow A. Diffuse alveolar damage. Am J Pathol 1976;85:210–228.
46. Pratt PC. Pathology of ARDS. In: The Lung: Structure, Function and Disease. Williams and Wilkins, 1978.
47. Knaus WA, Draper EA, Wagner DP, et al. Prognosis in acute organ system failure. Ann Surg 1985;202:685–691.
48. Montgomery AB, Stager MA, Carrico CF, et al. Causes of mortality in patients with ARDS. Am Rev Respir Dis 1985;132:485–489.
49. Hickling KG, Walsh J, Henderson S, et al. Low mortality rates in adult respiratory distress syndrome using low volume pressure limited ventilation with permissive hypercapnia: A prospective study. Crit Care Med 1994;22:1568–1578.
50. Castleman B. Case Records, Massachesetts General Hospital Clinicopatholgical Conference Case 33–1966. N Engl J Med 1966;V275:210–218.
51. Consentino AM. Pulmonary oxygen toxicity and machanical ventilation. N Engl J Med 1966;275:1078.
52. Morgan TE, Finley TN, Huber GL. Alterations in pulmonary surface active lipids during exposure to increased oxygen tension. J Clin Invest 1965;44: 1737–1744.
53. Nash G, Blennerhassett JB, Pontoppidan H. Pulmonary lesions associated with oxygen therapy and artificial ventilation. N Engl J Med 1967;276:368–374.
54. Webb HH, Tierney DF. Experimental pulmonary edema due to intermittent positive pressure ventilation with high inflation pressures. Protection by positive end-expiratory pressure. Am Rev Respir Dis 1974;110:556–565.
55. Singer MM, Wright F, Stanley L, et al. Oxygen toxicity in man: A prospective study in patients after heart surgery. N Engl J Med 1970;283:1473–1478.
56. Barber RE, Lee J, Hamilton WK. Oxygen toxicity in man: A prospective study in patients with irreversible brain damage. N Engl J Med 1970;283:1478–1484.
57. Deneke SM, Fanburg BL. Normobaric oxygen toxicity of the lung. Med Progress N Engl J Med 1980;303:76–86.
58. Gattinoni L, Tesanti A, Avalli L, et al. Pressure-volume curves of total respiratory system in acute respiratory failure. Computed tomographic scan study. Am Rev Respir Dis 1987;136:730–736.
59. Pelosi P, D'Andrea L, Vitale G, et al. Vertical gradient of regional lung inflation in ARDS. Am J Resp Crit Care Med 1994;149:8–13.
60. Muscedere JG, Mullen JBM, Gan K, et al. Tidal ventilation at low airway pressure can cause pulmonary barotrauma. Am J Respir Crit Care Med 1994;149: 1327–1334.
61. Bond DM, Froese AB. Volume recruitment maneuvers are less deleterious than persistant low lung volumes in the atelectasis prone rabbit lung during HFO. Crit Care Med 1993;21:402–412.
62. Boynton BR, Villanueva D, Hammond D, et al. Effect of mean airway pressure on gas exchange during HFOV. J Appl Physiol 1991;70:701–707.

63. Drazen JM, Kamm RD, Slatsky AS. High frequency ventilation. Physiol Rev 1984;64:505–543.
64. Walsh MC, Carlo WA. Sustained inflation during HFOV improves pulmonary mechanics and oxygenation. J Appl Physiol 1988;65:368–372.
65. The HIFI Study Group. HFOV compared with conventional mechanical ventilation in the treatment of respiratory failure in preterm infants. N Engl J Med 1989;320:88–93.
66. Dreyfuss D, Saumon G. Should the lung be rested or recruited? The charybdis and scylla of ventilator management. Am J Respir Crit Care Med 1994;149:1066–1068.
67. Lachmann B. Open the lung and keep the lung open. J Int Care Med 1992;18:319–321.
68. Suter PM, Fairley HB, Isenberg MD. Optimum end-expiratory pressure in patients with acute pulmonary failure. N Engl J Med 1975;292:284–289.
69. Tharratt RS, Allen RP, Albertson TE. Pressure controlled inverse ratio ventilation in severe ARDS. Chest 1988;94:755–762.
70. Lessard MR, Guerot E, Lorino H, et al. Effects of pressure controlled with different I:E ratios vs volume controlled ventilation in ARDS. Anesthesiology 1994;80:972–975.
71. Mercat A, Graini L, Teboul JL, et al. Cardio-respiratory effect of pressure controlled ventilation with and without inverse ratio in ARDS. Chest 1993;104:8871–8875.
72. Marini JJ. Ventilation of ARDS. Looking for Mr. Goodmode. Anesthesiology 1994;80:972–975.
73. Hickling KG, Walsh J, Henderson S, et al. Low mortality rates in adult respiratory distress syndrome using low volume pressure limited ventilation with permissive hypercapnia: A prospective study. Crit Care Med 1994;22:1568–1578.
74. Dreyfuss D, Soler P, Basset G, et al. High inflation pressure pulmonary edema. Respective effects of high airway pressure, high VT, and positive end-expiratory pressure. Am Rev Respir Dis 1988;137:1159–1164.
75. Dreyfuss D, Saumon G. Role of tidal volume, FRC, and inspiratory volume in the development of pulmonary edema following mechanical ventilation. Am Rev Respir Dis 1993;148:1194–1203.
76. Gattinoni H, Kolobow T, Tomlinson T, et al. Low frequency positive pressure ventilation and extra corporeal CO_2 removal. Anesth Analg 1978;55:470–477.
77. Nahum A, Burke WC, Ravenscraft SA, et al. Lung mechanics and gas exchange during pressure control ventilation in dogs: Augmentation of CO_2 elimination by an intratracheal catheter. Am Rev Respir Dis 1992;146:965–973.
78. Tutuncu AS, Faithfull NS, Lachmann B. Comparison of ventilatory support with intratracheal perfluorocarbon administration and conventional mechanical ventilation in animals with acute respiratory failure. Am Rev Respir Dis 1993;148:785–792.
79. Downs JB, Stock MC. Airway pressure release ventilation. Crit Care Med 1987;15:459–461.
80. Rasansen J, Cane RD, Downs JB, et al. APRV during acute lung injury. Crit Care Med 1991;19:1234–1241.
81. Springer RR, Stevens PM. Influence of PEEP on survival of patients in respiratory failure. Am J Med 1979;66:196–200.
82. Danek SJ, Lynch JP, Weg JG, et al. The dependence of oxygen uptake on oxygen delivery in the adult respiratory distress syndrome. Am Rev Respir Dis 1980;122:387–395.

83. Shoemaker WC, Appel PL, Kram HB, et al. Prospective trial of supranormal values of survivors as therapeutic goals in high risk surgical patients. Chest 1988;94:1176–1186.
84. Waxman K, Lazrove S, Shoemaker WC. Physiologic responses to operation in high risk surgical patients. Surg Gyn Obstet 1981;152:633–638.
85. Hayes MA, Timmins AC, Yau EHS, et al. Elevation of systemic oxygen delivery in the treatment of critically ill patients. N Engl J Med 1994;330:1717–1722.
86. Gattinoni H, Brazzi L, Pelosi P, et al. A trial of goal-oriented hemodynamic therapy in critically ill patients. N Engl J Med 1995;333:1025–1032.
87. Segredo V, Caldwell JE, Matthay M, et al. Persistent paralysis in critically ill patients after long term administration of Vecuronium. N Engl J Med 1992;327:524–528.
88. The Random House College Dictionary, Revised Edition. Random House, Inc., 1980, p. 1490.
89. Marin JJ (Chairman). Weaning from mechanical ventilation. American Thoracic Society Symposium. Am Rev Respir Dis 1988;138:1043–1046.
90. Brochard L, Rauss A, Benito S, et al. Comparison of three methods of gradual withdrawel from ventilatory support during weaning from mechanical ventilation. Am J Resp Crit Care Med 1994;150:896–903.
91. Esteban A, Frutos F, Tobin MJ. A comparison of four methods of weaning patients from mechanical ventilation. N Engl J Med 1995;332:345–350.
92. Yang KL, Tobin MJ. A prospective study of indexes predicting the outcome of trials of weaning from mechanical ventilation. N Engl J Med 1991;324:1445–1450.
93. Tobin MJ, Perez W, Guenther SM, et al. The pattern of breathing during successful and unsuccessful trials of weaning from mechanical ventilation. Am Rev Resp Dis 1986;134:1111–1118.
94. Sassoon CS, Light RW, Lodia R, et al. Pressure-time product during continuous positive airway pressure, pressure support ventilation, and T-piece during weaning from mechanical ventilation. Am Rev Resp Dis 1991;143:469–475.
95. The Random House College Dictionary, Revised Edition. Random House, Inc., 1980, p. 503.

Index

Please note: *t* refers to tabular content